DATE DUE

CHRONIC ANXIETY

CHRONIC ANXIETY
Generalized Anxiety Disorder
and
Mixed Anxiety–Depression

Editors

RONALD M. RAPEE
University of Queensland, Australia

DAVID H. BARLOW
University at Albany, State University of New York

THE GUILFORD PRESS
New York • London

© 1991 The Guilford Press
A Division of Guilford Publications, Inc.
72 Spring Street, New York, NY 10012

Printed in the United States of America

This book is printed on acid-free paper.

Last digit is print number: 9 8 7 6 5 4 3 2 1

Library of Congress Cataloging-in-Publication Data

Chronic anxiety : generalized anxiety disorder and mixed anxiety—
   depression / edited by Ronald M. Rapee, David H. Barlow.
      p. cm.
   Includes bibliographical references and index.
   ISBN 0-89862-771-0
   1. Anxiety.   2. Depression, Mental.   I. Rapee, Ronald M.
II. Barlow, David H.
   [DNLM: 1. Anxiety Disorders.   2. Depressive Disorder.   WM 172
C557]
RC531.C47   1991
616.85'223—dc20
DNLM/DLC
for Library of Congress   91-24737
                                                              CIP

Preface

The recognition of anxiety as one of the basic human emotions, and of disorders of anxiety as one of the foremost difficulties faced by humans, has a long history. Much of this history has been characterized by changes and improvements in the definition of subjects of anxiety-related problems. In recent years, one of the most influential developments in the conceptualization of the anxiety disorders came with the publication of the DSM-III. In this publication, official recognition was given to the hypothesis that nonspecific anxiety (anxiety without an obvious, immediate external trigger) came in two forms: panic attacks and generalized (chronic) anxiety. While a tremendous amount of research was subsequently generated into understanding the nature of panic attacks, generalized anxiety remained largely neglected.

It was because of this relative neglect that we felt the need to pull together a book reviewing the most up-to-date knowledge on chronic, generalized anxiety. We felt that chronic worry and generalized anxiety were fundamental aspects and common accompaniments to a broad range of psychopathology and, as such, greater understanding of these issues would have major implications not only for all of the anxiety disorders, but for a range of other disorders as well.

While compiling the chapters for the book, it became obvious that it would be impossible to adequately discuss chronic anxiety without also attending to the highly related and intertwined role of depressed mood. It was timely that at precisely this time the DSM-IV Anxiety Disorders Work Group was evaluating the possibility of including a new diagnostic category, Mixed Anxiety–Depression, to cover those individuals, many of whom present to general practitioners, who complain of equal mixtures of low levels of chronic anxiety and low mood. Since DHB chaired this Subgroup, we felt that it would round out the book to include some chapters devoted to the current deliberations in this area.

As suggested by the title, we have tried to include a combination of theoretical chapters that discuss some of the more fundamental constructs in addition to more clinical chapters devoted to discussing diagnosis, assessment, and treatment in the context of DSM categories. Thus, the book begins with a broad chapter describing a theoretical model of the emotional disorders and their interrelationships. The next three chapters aim at providing a fundamental understanding of worry and chronic anxiety, and, beginning with Chapter 5, the reader will find a more detailed examination of clinical issues.

Many of the chapters raise almost as many questions as they answer. In fact, this is a key focus of the book. Our main purpose in pulling together this group of authors was to raise consciousness about the importance of generalized anxiety and mixed anxiety–depression and, most importantly, to review the current state of knowledge in such a way that important directions for future research could be highlighted. Hopefully, these aims have been fulfilled and the coming years will see a marked increase in the acknowledged importance, understanding, and treatment of generalized anxiety and mixed anxiety–depression.

RONALD M. RAPEE
St. Lucia, Queensland

DAVID H. BARLOW
Nantucket Island
June 1991

Contributors

David H. Barlow, Ph.D., Department of Psychology, Center for Stress and Anxiety Disorders, University at Albany, State University of New York, Albany, New York

Aaron T. Beck, Ph.D., Center for Cognitive Therapy, University of Pennsylvania School of Medicine, Philadelphia, Pennsylvania

Richard G. Booth, Ph.D., Department of Psychology, University of British Columbia, Vancouver, Canada

Thomas D. Borkovec, Ph.D., The Stress and Anxiety Disorders Institute, Department of Psychology, Penn State University, University Park, Pennsylvania

Gillian Butler, Ph.D., Department of Psychology, Warneford Hospital, Headington, Oxford, UK

Deborah S. Cowley, M.D., Department of Psychiatry and Behavioral Sciences, University of Washington School of Medicine, Seattle, Washington

Peter A. Di Nardo, Ph.D., Center for Stress and Anxiety Disorders, University at Albany, State University of New York, Albany, New York, and State University College at Oneonta, Oneonta, New York

Bill Harman, M.A., Department of Psychology, George Mason University, Fairfax, Virginia

Ann A. Hohmann, Ph.D., National Institute of Mental Health, Bethesda, Maryland

Mildred Hopkins, M.S., The Stress and Anxiety Disorders Institute, Department of Psychology, Penn State University, University Park, Pennsylvania

Roger Moore, M.A., Department of Psychology, George Mason University, Fairfax, Virginia

Ronald M. Rapee, Ph.D., Department of Psychology, University of Queensland, St. Lucia, Queensland, Australia

Karl Rickels, M.D., Psychopharmacology Research Unit, Department of Psychiatry, University of Pennsylvania/University Hospital, Philadelphia, Pennsylvania

John Riskind, M.D., Department of Psychology, George Mason University, Fairfax, Virginia

Peter P. Roy-Byrne, M.D., Department of Psychiatry and Behavioral Sciences, University of Washington School of Medicine, Seattle, Washington

William C. Sanderson, Ph.D., Department of Psychiatry, Albert Einstein College of Medicine/Montefiore Medical Center, Bronx, New York

Edward Schweizer, M.D., Psychopharmacology Research Unit, Department of Psychiatry, University of Pennsylvania/University Hospital, Philadelphia, Pennsylvania

Richard N. Shadick, M.S., The Stress and Anxiety Disorders Institute, Department of Psychology, Penn State University, University Park, Pennsylvania

Bonnie Stewart, M.A., Center for Cognitive Therapy, University of Pennsylvania School of Medicine, Philadelphia, Pennsylvania

Scott Wetzler, Ph.D., Department of Psychiatry, Albert Einstein College of Medicine/Montefiore Medical Center, Bronx, New York

Richard E. Zinbarg, Ph.D., Center for Stress and Anxiety Disorders, University at Albany, State University of New York, Albany, New York

Contents

1

The Nature of Anxiety: Anxiety, Depression, and Emotional Disorders

DAVID H. BARLOW
University at Albany, State University of New York

T he purposes of this chapter are to review accumulated knowledge on anxiety and to present a new model of emotional disorders. Central to this model is a theory of the relationship of anxiety and "neurotic" depression; it is suggested that these are fundamentally similar or identical affective states, with neurotic depression being the chronologically later and more severe expression of anxiety. After individual models of anxiety and depression are described, and the relationship of panic attacks and discrete bouts of endogenous depression to anxiety and neurotic depression is outlined, the model of emotional disorders is presented. The chapter ends with conclusions on the importance of gaining a deeper understanding of anxiety if we are to advance in our ability to diagnose and treat emotional disorders.

TRADITIONS IN THE STUDY OF ANXIETY

Theories of anxiety have proliferated and can be categorized, roughly, as behavioral, biological, or cognitive. The behavioral approach is best represented by the discrete-emotion theorists, who highlight a neoevolutionary approach continuing the tradition of Darwin (1872). In this tradition, emotions are innate, "hard-wired" patterns of reaction and responding that have evolved in many life forms because of their functional significance. For example, the purpose of the fear reaction is motivation to escape from imminent danger (the flight part of the fight–flight reaction). In addition, the basic emotion of fear is fundamentally distinct from other basic emotions

1

such as sadness/distress or anger. Discrete emotions play a role in my model of anxiety disorders and other emotional disorders as presented below.

Izard (1977) and Izard and Blumberg (1985), who best represent the expressive behavioral approach, view anxiety as a hybrid or blend of a number of basic emotions, although fear is admittedly dominant in the blend. The basic emotions most commonly considered to combine with fear to make up anxiety include distress/sadness, anger, shame, guilt, and interest/excitement. Furthermore, anxiety, according to Izard's view, may assume a different blend across time and situations. For example, in one instance fear, distress, and anger may be the blend referred to as "anxiety" by the individual; in another instance shame and guilt may be combined with fear. Naturally, such combinations make it very difficult to talk of anxiety in a precise way in the behavioral tradition. Furthermore, each of the fundamental innate emotions is modified by learning and experience. Individuals may learn to associate discrete emotions such as fear with a large number of cognitive and situational factors, including the evocation of other, related emotions.

Theorists of all persuasions admit to the role of neurobiology in anxiety, but some consider it primary and causal (see Chapter 3 for current thinking on the biology of anxiety). Current neurobiological models of anxiety, which trace their heritage back to Cannon (1929), emphasize the trait-like nature of anxiety and the origins of these traits in the brain. Perhaps the best-known theorists from this point of view are Eysenck (1981), Gray (1982), and most recently, Cloninger (1986). All of these theories posit specific neuroanatomical regions of the brain and specific neurotransmitter systems as underlying anxious responding. For example, in Cloninger's theorizing, which relies heavily on the prior thinking of Gray and Eysenck, anxiety (or high harm avoidance) is associated with high serotonergic activity (see Barlow, 1988, for a review).

A relatively recent development is the notion of anxiety as cognition, best represented in the writings of Richard Lazarus (1968), Charles Spielberger (1985), and, most recently, Aaron T. Beck (e.g., Beck, Emery, & Greenberg, 1985). Although these theories differ considerably in detail, they are fundamentally attribution or appraisal theories, wherein the perceiving organism appraises certain aspects of the environment as dangerous and reacts accordingly. This appraisal most often occurs after an interruption of some sort. Appraisals result in a variety of negative and fearful cognitive processes, which are sometimes thought to predate the specific appraisal (e.g., Beck et al., 1985).

Most recently, the bioinformational theory of Peter Lang has emerged as an important model of anxiety. Although it is most easily classified as a cognitive theory, Lang's model does not depend on conscious (or unconscious) appraisals, but rather on the activation of various cognitive processes stored in memory. Fear in this model is a very focused and specific memory network, whereas anxiety is more diffuse and vague. Lang's model (1979, 1984, 1985) has a great deal of heuristic value and has deeply influenced my own model of anxiety, presented below.

A MODEL OF ANXIETY

As noted above, most emotion theorists who have addressed the issue have concluded that anxiety is a construct that differs from related emotions such as anger and fear. Evidence supporting the distinction between anxiety and fear is presented below.

On the basis of data developed in our center and elsewhere, as well as the theories and traditions described above, I think that the evidence supports a conceptualization of anxiety as a loose cognitive–affective structure. This construct is composed primarily of high negative affect, associated with a sense of uncontrollability, and a shift in attention to a focus primarily on the self or a state of self-preoccupation. The sense of uncontrollability is focused on future threat, danger, or other negative events. Thus, this negative affective state can be characterized roughly as a state of "helplessness" because of perceived inabilities to predict, control, or obtain desired results in certain upcoming situations or contexts. If one were to put anxiety into words, one might say, "That terrible event is not my fault but it may happen again, and I may not be able to cope with it but I've got to be ready to try." From this point of view, a better and more precise term for "anxiety" might be "anxious apprehension." This conveys the notion that anxiety is a future-oriented mood state in which one is ready or prepared to attempt to cope with upcoming negative events. This is best reflected in the state of chronic overarousal that seems to characterize anxiety and those who present with anxiety. This arousal may be the physiological substrate of "readiness," which may underlie an effort to counteract helplessness (e.g., Fridlund, Hatfield, Cottam, & Fowler, 1986). Vigilance (hypervigilance) is another characteristic of anxiety that suggests readiness and preparation to deal with negative events. The process of anxiety, as this model would have it, is presented in Figure 1.1.

With more specific reference to Figure 1.1, a variety of cues (or "propositions," in Lang's [1985] terms) may be sufficient to evoke anxious apprehension without the necessity of a conscious, rational appraisal. The cues may be broad-based or very narrow, as in the case of test anxiety or sexual dysfunction. The state of negative affect, with its associated arousal

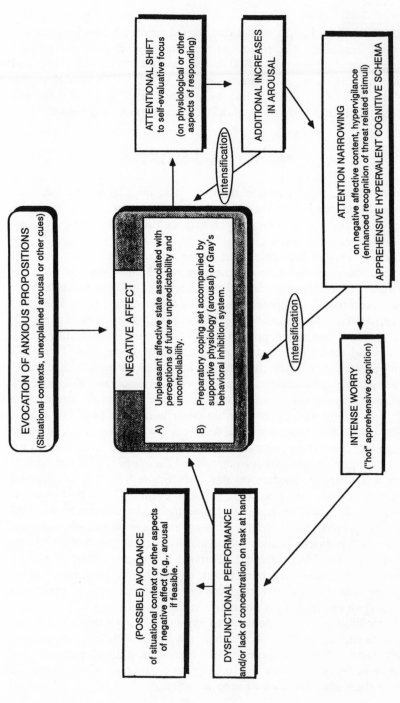

FIGURE 1.1. The process of anxious apprehension. From *Anxiety and Its Disorders: The Nature and Treatment of Anxiety and Panic* by D. H. Barlow, 1988, New York: The Guilford Press. Copyright 1988 by The Guilford Press. Reprinted by permission.

and negative valence, is in turn associated with distortions in information processing. These cognitive distortions are characterized by an attentional shift to a self-evaluative focus (or a rapidly shifting focus of attention from external sources to internal self-evaluative content).

The importance of self-focused attention has been underestimated in theories of negative affect. It has been clear for some time that individuals can be highly proficient at discriminating changes in autonomic activity (e.g., Schwartz, 1976). Nevertheless, as Shapiro (1974) points out, the relatively poor utilization of this potential may have been functionally adaptive in an evolutionary sense. That is, placing a limit on awareness of internal events reduces an important source of distraction to ongoing external activity.

Several aspects of the work on self-focused attention are relevant to a theory of anxiety. First, self-focused attention greatly increases sensitivity to bodily sensations and other sources of internal experience. Second, this sensitivity to bodily sensations quickly spreads to other aspects of the self, such as self-evaluative concerns (Carver & Scheier, 1981; Scheier, Carver, & Matthews, 1983). Furthermore, this self-directed focus and the resulting increased sensitivity to physiological or proprioceptive sensations are likely to result in greater subjective intensity of emotional experience. One additional important consequence of self-focused attention is a failure to habituate to external stimuli while in this attentional mode (Scheier et al., 1983). This aspect of self-focused attention has substantial implications for theories of anxiety reduction. Thus, in Figure 1.1 self-focused attention is represented as further increasing arousal, forming its own small positive feedback loop with negative affect. This condition is particularly salient if the direction of self-attention is allocated to the affective qualities of the experience, and particularly if the affect is negative (Scheier et al., 1983).

The arousal and activation associated with this process lead to a dramatic narrowing of attention to the content of the apprehension, as well as self-preoccupation with one's ability to obtain desired results in the upcoming situation(s). It is not arousal per se that is problematic in this process, since an external focus of attention and a sense of control combined with arousal may well produce effective performance. Rather, essential to this process are the arousal-driven apprehension and self-preoccupation. Extreme arousal, whatever the cause, will eventually result in deterioration of attention and performance (Korchin, 1964).

Hypervigilance, or the enhanced recognition of threat-related stimuli (MacLeod, Mathews, & Tata, 1986), is one consequence of attention narrowing. But hypervigilance will be directed differently, depending on the perceived source of threat. For example, in sexual dysfunction any signs of demands for sexual performance will trigger anxious apprehension, leading to attention narrowing and hypervigilance to these cues. Similarly, simple phobics will be hypervigilant for environmental cues that provide a context for feared objects or situations. Sartory (1986) has confirmed the hypervigilance of simple phobics with fears of small animals to environmental stimuli. On the other hand, research from a variety of sources has highlighted the hypervigilance of patients with panic disorder to internal somatic cues that may signal the beginning of the next panic attack.

In its extreme state, narrowing of attention of apprehensive concerns leads to runaway, out-of-control, intense worry that individuals are unable to shut off or control in any effective way. Worry in turn leads to disruptions in concentration, which constitute one of the hallmarks of clinical anxiety; these are accompanied by disruptions in performance, if performance is required. In sexual or test-taking contexts, disruptions in performance become the most salient part of the problem. When anxiety is generalized, difficulties in concentration may lead to inefficient performance at the job or at home, but patients place more emphasis on the unpleasantness associated with chronic, unremitting states of anxious apprehension. Attempts to avoid a negative affective state are inevitable, but may not be successful. Avoidance may fail because of the diffuseness of the cues or because of the necessity of encountering the situation or context even if the cues are very restricted, as is the case with most individuals suffering from test anxiety. (For a more detailed description of research on the process of worry, see Chapter 2 of this volume.)

At sufficient intensity, this process results in disruption of concentration and performance, and ultimately in avoidance of sources of apprehension (if this method of coping is available). Arousal-driven anxious apprehension will, of course, only interfere with performance if some performance is required. In situations where performance may not be called for immediately, but where perceptions of loss of control or other negative affective content have become associated with a number of important life events (e.g., health, finances, and family concerns), then the process of worry will emerge. The intensity of worry will increase or decrease, depending on situational context, the amount of underlying autonomic arousal that is available at the time for transfer (Zillmann, 1983), and/or the presence of other "propositions" capable of calling forth this diffuse cognitive–affective structure.

More detailed evidence for each of these components of anxiety and their connection is presented in some detail elsewhere (Barlow, 1988). It is also important to note that this is not a description of the etiology of anxiety but rather an illustration of the process of anxious apprehension. The etiology of anxious apprehension, and the biological and psychological vulnerabilities that predispose individuals to this state, are described below and fully discussed elsewhere (Barlow, 1988).

What is the purpose of anxiety? Why are we programmed to become anxious? This has prompted much speculation from philosophers and psychologists, but also some data. We have known for over 80 years that organisms become more vigilant, learn more quickly, and perform better both motorically and intellectually if anxious (Yerkes & Dobson, 1908). We also know that both benzodiazepines and relaxation interfere with effective performance (Barlow, 1988). From this point of view, anxiety can be very adaptive (up to a point), and the adaptive purpose of anxiety would seem to be planning and preparation to meet a challenge or threat. As Howard Liddell (1949) noted,

> The planning function of the nervous system, in the course of evolution, has culminated in the appearance of ideas, values, and pleasures—the unique manifestations of man's social living. Man, alone, can plan for the distant future and can experience the retrospective pleasures of achievement. Man, alone, can be happy. But man, alone, can be worried and anxious. Sherrington once said that posture accompanies movement as a shadow. I have come to believe that anxiety accompanies intellectual activity as its shadow and that the more we know of the nature of anxiety, the more we will know of intellect. (p. 185)

It is also well known that anxiety is distributed as a trait (Eysenck, 1967, 1981) and is expressed more or less by most individuals under certain situations. Therefore, it is only very intense anxiety—or perhaps anxiety with an inappropriate focus—that comes to the attention of clinicians. In addition, as noted above, strong evidence supports the existence of both biological and psychological vulnerabilities to developing anxiety. I return to these vulnerabilities below.

A MODEL OF DEPRESSION

What is depression, and how does it differ from anxiety? Many different points of view on this distinction have appeared (e.g., Kendall & Watson, 1989). A number of theorists have concluded that anxiety and depression are variable expressions of the same pathology. Yet another group of theorists supposes that anxiety and depression are fundamentally different and distinct. Other theorists fall somewhere in between, suggesting, for example, a common diathesis with subsequent divergence occurring for any one of a number of reasons (Weissman, 1985).

The evidence for a unitary view is very strong. For example, on a neurobiological level the process seems to be very similar or perhaps identical. Gray (1985), reviewing evidence from the animal laboratories, suggests that learned helplessness (construed as an animal model of depression) may be identical in its neurobiological underpinnings to models of anxiety.

Specifically, enhanced hippocampal function as a result of increased nor-adrenergic input to this and other regions of the forebrain seem to underlie both anxiety and depression. Interestingly, Breier, Charney, and Heninger (1985) found identical, greatly enhanced underlying noradrenergic activity in clinical populations with either panic disorder or major depressive disorder.

Several recent studies have also shown that patients with relatively pure cases of generalized anxiety disorder or panic disorder show similar rates of nonsuppression on the dexamethasone suppression test when com-pared to cases of major depression (e.g., Schweizer, Swenson, Winokur, Rickels, & Maislin, 1986; Coryell, Noyes, Clancy, Crowe, & Chaudhry, 1985; Avery et al., 1985), although other studies without depressive control groups show that panickers are not significantly different from normals on this test (e.g., Roy-Byrne, Bierer, & Uhde, 1985).

In addition to this evidence, data from family studies strongly suggest that anxiety, depression, and panic are closely related. Generally, the more signs and symptoms of anxiety and depression, the greater the rate of anxiety or depression or both in first-degree relatives and children (Puig-Antich & Rabinovich, 1986; Weissman, 1985; Leckman, Weissman, Mer-ikangas, Pauls, & Prusoff, 1983).

Finally, the emerging evidence from pharmacological treatments for both anxiety and depressive disorders is that tricyclic antidepressants seem to be the treatment of choice. Although these drugs are known as "anti-depressants," it now seems clear that they are effective with anxiety disorders such as panic disorder, and not just for panic disorder with accompanying depression (Mavissakalian & Michelson, 1986; Mavissakalian, 1987). Fur-thermore, evidence now exists that tricyclics such as imipramine are effective with anxiety disorders in which panic is not a prominent feature, such as generalized anxiety disorder (Kahn, Stevenson, Topol, & Klein, 1986; Klein, Rabkin, & Gorman, 1985; see Chapter 9). In addition, a close analysis of the literature suggests that the effectiveness of tricyclics in cases of panic disorder may *not* necessarily be due to direct blockade of panic, as commonly assumed; rather, it may be due to therapeutic effects on anxious apprehension associated with panic (Barlow, 1988). There is also evidence that new high-potency benzodiazepines such as alprazolam are effective not only for panic disorder (Ballenger et al., 1988), but also for some types of depressive disorders (e.g., Rickels, Feighner, & Smith, 1985). Thus, evidence from both basic neurobiological studies and drug treatment studies exists that supports the unitary view of anxiety and depression. Of course, evidence also exists supporting different biological processes associated with at least some presentations of anxiety and depression (Roy-Byrne, Mellman, & Uhde, 1988; see Chapter 3). Clarification may have to await more precise subtyping or new models of this relationship of anxiety and depression, such as that presented below.

Do questionnaires and inventories provide any help in discriminating anxiety and depression? In fact, an examination of popular rating scales for either anxiety or depression demonstrates that whether one is measuring anxiety or depression, these scales correlate very highly. For example, Dobson (1985) examined scales such as the State–Trait Anxiety Inventory (Spielberger, Gorsuch, & Lushene, 1970) and the Zung Self-Rating Depression Scale (Zung, 1965), among others. The correlation among anxiety scales was .66; among depression scales it was .69; and among anxiety and depression scales it was .61. The amount of shared variance for each correlation was very high, ranging from .37 to .48. This degree of shared variance suggests that these questionnaires are not useful in measuring the intensity of two different affective states, anxiety and depression; rather, they are measuring the same or very similar affective states. This reflects a finding also reported by Gotlieb (1984)—namely, that self-report measures of depression and anxiety correlated highly in college students (see Gotlieb & Cane, 1989) for a thorough discussion of this issue).

Do clinical rating scales discriminate between anxiety and depression? The most popular and widely used rating scales for anxiety and depression are the Hamilton scales (Hamilton, 1959, 1960). But on these scales the overlap on specific questions exceeds 70% (Barlow, 1985). Therefore it is not surprising that these scales are highly correlated, share considerable variance, and demonstrate poor discriminant validity. For example, groups with depressive diagnoses score as high as or higher than any anxiety disorder group on the Hamilton Anxiety Rating Scale (Di Nardo & Barlow, 1990). Similarly, many anxiety disorders do not differ significantly from depressive disorders on the Hamilton Rating Scale for Depression. Of course, discriminant validity or diagnosis is not the purpose of these scales.

Nevertheless, in our clinic since the early 1980s, we have identified several items from the Hamilton scales that seem to discriminate anxious and depressed clients consistently (Barlow, 1983). Primary among these items, in addition to suicidal thoughts and depressed mood, are feelings of hopelessness and motor retardation. These findings are presented in Table 1.1. This finding is not unique to our clinic, but has been reported since the 1950s by Sir Martin Roth and colleagues (e.g., Roth, Gurney, Garside, & Kerr, 1972).

More recently, Riskind, Beck, Brown, and Steer (1987) revised the two Hamilton scales to discriminate more clearly between anxiety and depressive disorders in clinical populations. This revision is one of the first attempts to construct scales based on what is essential and important about anxiety and depression when compared to each other, as opposed to scale construction based simply on descriptors of unpleasant mood or dysphoria that are common to both anxiety and depression. Items were reassigned

TABLE 1.1. Hamilton Depression Items for Different Diagnostic Groups

	Agoraphobia	Social phobia	Simple phobia	Panic disorder	GAD	Obsessive compulsive	Major affective
Retardation	1.09_a	1.13_a	1.00_a	1.00_a	1.00_a	1.25_a	1.58_b
Suicide	1.55_b	1.50_{ab}	1.36_{ab}	1.18_a	1.13_a	1.33_{ab}	2.33_c
Helplessness	1.79_a	1.55_a	1.57_a	1.58_a	1.45_a	2.00_a	2.67_b

Note. Means with similar subscripts are not significantly different. GAD, generalized anxiety disorder. From Barlow, D. H. (1983, October). *The classification of anxiety disorders.* Paper presented at the conference DSM-III: An Interim Appraisal, sponsored by the American Psychiatric Association, Washington, DC.

TABLE 1.2. Comparison of Anxiety Disorder and Depressed Groups on Revised Hamilton Scales

Scale	Simple phobia (n = 20)	Social phobia (n = 19)	Major depression (n = 15)	Dysthymia (n = 15)	GAD (n = 20)	OCD (n = 17)	Panic disorder (n = 19)	Mixed (n = 19)	Agoraphobia with panic (n = 18)
Anxiety	17.3_a	19.3_{ab}	20.3_{abc}	21.0_{bcd}	21.2_{bcd}	23.4_{cd}	23.7_{de}	25.3_{ef}	27.1_f
Depression	16.3_a	19.9_{bc}	29.9_f	28.9_f	20.3_{bcd}	24.4_{de}	20.2_{bc}	23.9_{de}	22.6_{de}

Note. Means with identical subscripts are not significantly different (at .05 level). GAD, generalized anxiety disorder; OCD, obsessive compulsive disorder. The data are from McCauley, Di Nardo, and Barlow (1987) and Di Nardo and Barlow (1990).

after factor analyses and point-biserial correlational analyses, based on scores from relatively pure groups of anxious and depressed patients without comorbid depressive or anxiety diagnoses. As a result of this analysis, all items associated with arousal or activation were reassigned to the Hamilton Anxiety Rating Scale (Riskind et al., 1987). From this point of view fundamental differences between clearly defined anxiety and depression may be found in action tendencies and underlying associated physiology. "Pure" anxiety suggests engagement and activation; "pure" depression suggests disengagement and inactivity. Anxiety implies an effort to cope with difficult situations, and the physiology is there to support active attempts at coping. Depression is characterized by behavioral retardation and an associated lack of arousal. With this clarification, we can also bid farewell to the conceptually muddled concept of "agitated depression." Agitation clearly groups with activation and chronic overarousal, which are at the core of anxiety. This contrasts with motor retardation and loss of pleasurable engagement, which are characteristics unique to depression.

Nevertheless, even with these revisions, revised Hamilton scores reflect the fact that patients earning a diagnosis of depression are anxious. We now have two different samples of anxiety disorder patients from our clinic to whom we have administered these revised Hamilton scales (McCauley, Di Nardo, & Barlow, 1987; Di Nardo & Barlow, 1990). Table 1.2 shows that the patients with depressive disorders are no longer the most anxious on the Hamilton Anxiety Rating Scale, but they are still more "anxious" than those with simple or social phobia. However, on the Hamilton Rating Scale for Depression, the patients with depressive disorders are now clearly significantly different from all patients with anxiety disorders.

These developments also underscore the value of studying relatively pure groups of patients in an effort to uncover the nature of anxiety and depression. We have now begun this investigation along several lines. In one study we compared the attributions of dysthymic patients to those of normal controls. To these groups we compared the attributions of anxiety patients who were arrayed on the Beck Depression Inventory (BDI, which contains ratings of the intensity of core depressive symptoms) as either nondepressed or moderately depressed. Nevertheless, no anxiety disorder patients, even those scoring in the moderately depressed range on the BDI, received an additional depressive disorder diagnosis. Attributions were assessed by the well-known Attributional Style Questionnaire (Peterson et al., 1982). The results indicated clear differences between anxious and depressed patients *once the presence and severity of depressive symptoms were controlled for by covariation procedures.* That is, depressed patients displayed internal, global, and stable attributions for negative outcomes. Some anxiety patients also demonstrated this attributional style, *but only if they were also depressed.* Anxiety patients, despite the severity of their anxiety disorder, had scores almost identical to those of the normal group if they were not depressed (Heimberg, Vermilyea, Dodge, Becker, & Barlow, 1987). In fact, cognitive content (particularly depressive cognitive content), but *not* cognitive processes, seems a reasonably good way to discriminate relatively pure cases of anxiety and depression (Kendall & Watson, 1989; see also Chapter 8, this volume).

Thus, scores on rating scales as well as our study of attributional style tend to converge on one conclusion: Signs and symptoms of depression, but *not* signs and symptoms of anxiety, discriminate these groups. To put it in another way, almost all depressed patients are anxious, but not all anxious patients are depressed. Evidence from a variety of other sources and methods, in studies with both adults and children, also reflects this general conclusion. For example, a close examination of patterns of co-morbidity in our clinic suggests that individuals presenting with anxiety disorders do not necessarily present with comorbid depressive diagnoses, but clients with diagnosable depressive disorders very often present with comorbid anxiety diagnoses (Barlow, Di Nardo, Vermilyea, Vermilyea, & Blanchard, 1986; Di Nardo & Barlow, 1990; Barlow, 1988; Sanderson, Di Nardo, Rapee, & Barlow, 1990).

This general conclusion is also supported when one examines the broad mood factors of negative and positive affect, as isolated by Auke Tellegen (1985) and presented in Figure 1.2. For example, Watson, Clark, and Carey (1988), working within this framework, found that negative affect correlated broadly with symptoms and diagnoses of both anxiety and depression. But positive affect was related (negatively) only to symptoms and diagnoses of depression, indicating that the loss of pleasurable engagement or anhedonia, which is the hallmark of low positive affect, is a distinctive feature of depression (see also Watson & Kendall, 1989). This information, along with the frequent observation that anxiety tends to precede the occurrence of depressive episodes, suggests one possible general conclusion: At least certain types of depression are later complications of anxiety occurring in some people under some conditions.

THE CAUSES OF ANXIETY AND DEPRESSION

A detailed discussion of etiology is not possible in the context of this chapter, but I have suggested elsewhere (Barlow, 1988) that anxiety and depression share a common biological vulnerability, best described as an overactive neurobiological response to stressful life events. This would be conceptualized as a general tendency to develop anxiety (or depression),

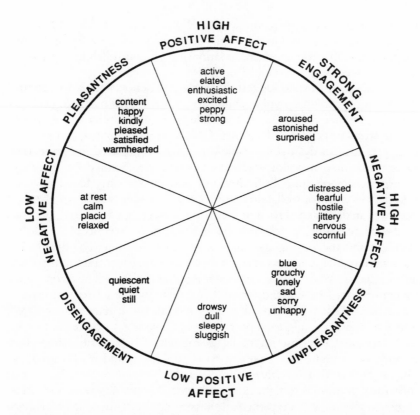

FIGURE 1.2. The two-factor structure of self-rated mood. From "Structures of Mood and Personality and Their Relevance to Assessing Anxiety, with an Emphasis on Self-Report," by A. Tellegen, in *Anxiety and the Anxiety Disorders* (p. 691) edited by A. H. Tuma and J. D. Maser, 1985, Hillsdale, NJ: Erlbaum. Copyright 1985 by Lawrence Erlbaum Associates. Reprinted by permission.

rather than a specific vulnerability for anxiety or depression itself. In addition to this biological vulnerability, I have also suggested that these individuals possess a psychological vulnerability based on early experiences with controllability. Here the pioneering work of Susan Mineka in reinterpreting the importance of the variable of uncontrollability in some of the early experimental neurosis work is extremely relevant (Mineka, 1985a, 1985b; Mineka & Kihlstrom, 1978). More recent work, elucidating the effects in primates of early experiences with uncontrollability on later manifestations of fear and anxiety is also crucial (Mineka, Gunnar, & Champoux, 1986). In fact, the concept of control or lack of it has an important history in psychology, as is evident in the work of Julian Rotter (1954) and George Mandler (1966), as well as in Martin Seligman's (1975) work on learned helplessness. But somehow the relationship of controllability to anxiety seems to have been overlooked until its recent revival.

In any case, I would suggest that early experiences with lack of control provide a psychological vulnerability for anxiety. This psychological vulnerability, when combined with a biological vulnerability and triggered by the stress of negative life events, leads to clinical anxiety, and possibly to depression (or dysthymia) some time later (as depicted in Figure 1.3). Depression, then, may simply reflect an extreme psychological vulnerability to experiences of unpredictability and uncontrollability, based on early experiences with controllability and coping. In other words, whether one becomes anxious and stays that way, or also becomes depressed, depends on the extent of one's psychological vulnerability, the severity of the current stressor, and the coping mechanisms at one's disposal. The greater the vulnerability, the more severe the stressor, and the fewer the coping mechanisms that are available, the more likely it is that anxiety will be accompanied by depression. I have noted above that one might put anxiety into words by saying, "That terrible event is not my fault but it may happen again, and I may not be able to cope with it but I've got to be ready to try." The depressed response might be as follows: "That terrible event may happen again and I won't be able to cope with it, and it's probably my fault anyway so there's really nothing I can do." In other words, the anxious individual continues to fight the good fight, but the depressed individual begins to give up. What is particularly interesting about this conceptualization is that Lauren Alloy, Susan Mineka, and their students, coming at it from the viewpoint of hopelessness depression, have arrived at essentially the same conclusion as depicted in Figure 1.4.

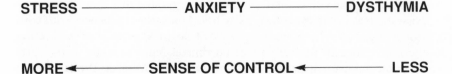

FIGURE 1.3. Proposed relationship of a sense of control to states of anxiety and depression (dysthymia).

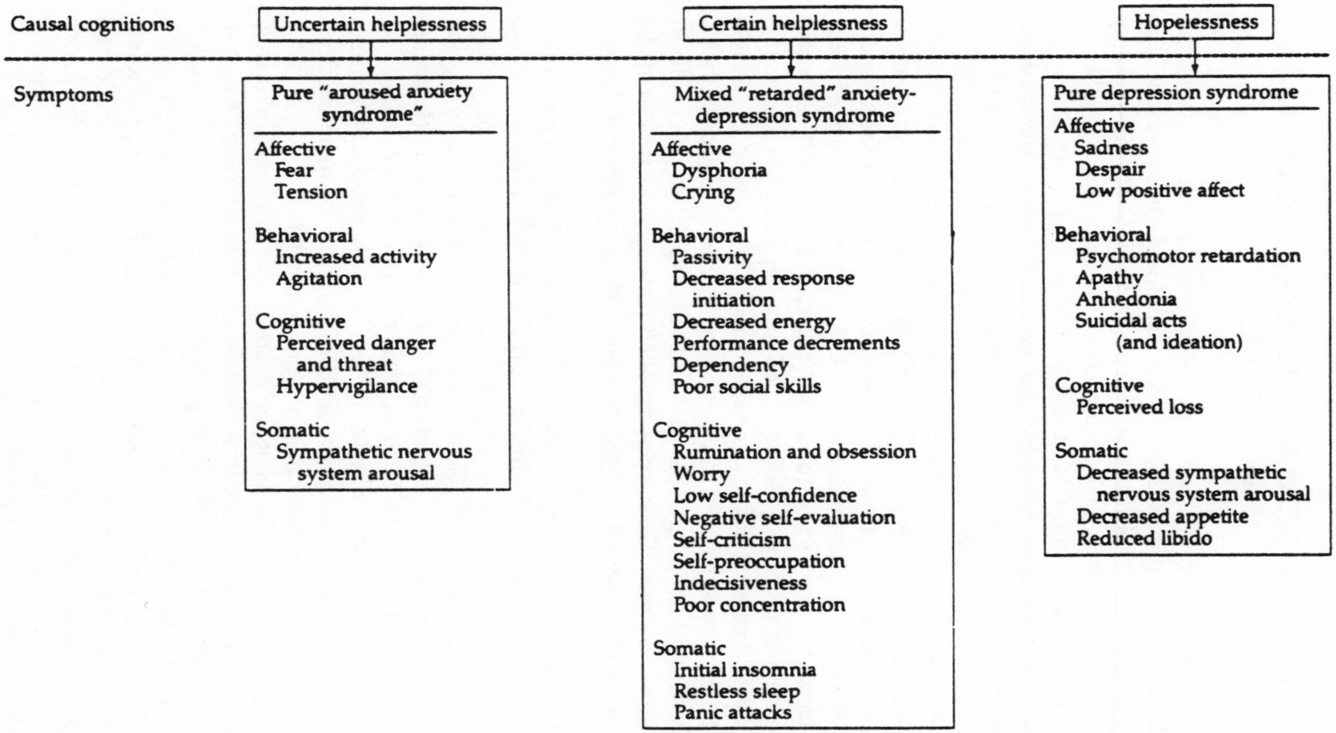

Causal cognitions	Uncertain helplessness	Certain helplessness	Hopelessness
Symptoms	Pure "aroused anxiety syndrome"	Mixed "retarded" anxiety-depression syndrome	Pure depression syndrome

Pure "aroused anxiety syndrome"

Affective
Fear
Tension

Behavioral
Increased activity
Agitation

Cognitive
Perceived danger and threat
Hypervigilance

Somatic
Sympathetic nervous system arousal

Mixed "retarded" anxiety-depression syndrome

Affective
Dysphoria
Crying

Behavioral
Passivity
Decreased response initiation
Decreased energy
Performance decrements
Dependency
Poor social skills

Cognitive
Rumination and obsession
Worry
Low self-confidence
Negative self-evaluation
Self-criticism
Self-preoccupation
Indecisiveness
Poor concentration

Somatic
Initial insomnia
Restless sleep
Panic attacks

Pure depression syndrome

Affective
Sadness
Despair
Low positive affect

Behavioral
Psychomotor retardation
Apathy
Anhedonia
Suicidal acts (and ideation)

Cognitive
Perceived loss

Somatic
Decreased sympathetic nervous system arousal
Decreased appetite
Reduced libido

FIGURE 1.4. Symptom predictions of the hopelessness theory. From Alloy, L. B., Kelly, K. A., Mineka, S., & Clements, C. M. (1990). Comorbidity in anxiety and depressive disorders: A helplessness–hopelessness perspective. In J. D. Maser & C. R. Cloninger (Eds.), *Comorbidity of mood and anxiety disorders.* Washington, DC: American Psychiatric Press. Copyright 1990 by American Psychiatric Press. Reprinted with permission.

15

PANIC, ENDOGENOUS DEPRESSION, FEAR, AND SADNESS

Within the anxiety disorders, one of the most profound developments in the past decade in terms of its impact on research and clinical practice has been the emergence of the phenomenon of panic. Panic attacks are typically described as sudden bursts of emotion consisting of a large number of somatic symptoms and thoughts of dying and/or losing control. On the average, these symptoms are relatively consistent across people experiencing panic; however, individual panic attacks may present with a different "mix" or number of symptoms and may vary in intensity. A prominent feature of many of these attacks as they present in the clinic is the report by the client, at least initially, that no frightening situation or thought process (cue) was associated with the attack. Clients may also report the attack to be totally unexpected. Although the uncued, unexpected nature of panic attacks is clearly a construct of the client (i.e., cues are usually discovered after a systematic examination; Barlow, 1988), this phenomenon has resulted in the labeling of these attacks as "spontaneous." Of course, panic attacks may also be expected and have cues, as in the case of the specific phobic who is afraid to cross bridges (the cue) and fully expects to panic if he or she must cross a bridge. These cued expected panic attacks are essentially similar in their presentation to "spontaneous" attacks (Barlow & Craske, 1990).

What is panic? I have argued elsewhere (Barlow, 1988, in press) that panic has many similarities to the emotion of fear. Emotion theorists generally agree that fear is a distinct, primitive, basic emotion, or perhaps a tightly organized, cohesive affective structure stored in memory, and that it is fundamentally a behavioral act. Fear is associated with intense neurobiological and cognitive features. Fear occurs when we are directly and imminently threatened—whether by wild animals, which was so often the case when our distant ancestors lived in caves, or by more modern-day dangers, such as a vehicle careening out of control.

The action tendency that is at the heart of this emotion is the well-known fight-or-flight response. It is essential that this response be instantaneous, since the survival of the organism may depend on it. This is Cannon's (1929) emergency response or alarm reaction. Most theorists would agree that this response is evolutionarily favored, ancient, and found far down the phylogenetic scale. Subjectively, the response is characterized by an overwhelming urge to escape, most often expressed as "I've got to get out of here." This would seem to reflect the basic action tendency of escape. What is the clinical manifestation of fear? Accumulating developmental and phenomenological evidence would seem to indicate that panic attacks represent the clinical manifestation of the basic emotion of fear. The hairtrigger, instantaneous quality of fear is very well illustrated in panic attacks captured serendipitously in the laboratory. In one case (Cohen, Barlow, & Blanchard, 1985), we found that an unexpected surge of autonomic arousal with accompanying subjective manifestations of fear peaked and then diminished substantially in the space of 3 minutes.

PANIC VERSUS ANXIETY

In addition to the evidence reviewed above, there are a number of reasons to believe that panic, as a clinical manifestation of fear, is best conceptualized as distinct from anxiety. First, both physiological and phenomenological evidence suggests that panic attacks are descriptively and functionally unique events when compared to anxiety. Panic attacks present differently from anxious apprehension and are experienced differently by clients (Barlow et al., 1985; Cohen et al., 1985; Rapee, 1985; Taylor et al., 1986). Second, research demonstrating a strong functional relationship between panic attacks and subsequent anticipatory anxiety is now appearing (e.g., Rachman & Levitt, 1985). That is, whether a panic attack occurs or not in a specific circumstance and whether it is expected or not will influence subsequent anxiety (and avoidance) associated with the phobic situation. In this regard, it is conceptually difficult to consider the alternative of developing "anxiety" focused on the future experience of "anxiety." Third, a strong (although not universal) consensus from the basic study of emotion, as noted above, suggests a fundamental difference between anxiety and fear. Fear is thought to be a basic action tendency of fight or flight that is a tightly organized affective structure in memory. This contrasts with anxiety, which is seen as a blend of basic emotions or, more likely, as a diffuse cognitive–affective structure associated with preparation for future threat or challenge. Unlike biological models of panic, this hypothetical separation of anxiety and panic does *not* imply that panic itself involves a biological dysregulation. Rather, panic is conceptualized as a normal fear response firing inappropriately.

Further circumstantial evidence for this conceptual separation is present in genetic studies and studies of the aggregation of emotion-related action tendencies. Although family studies of panic in clinical context have been confounded somewhat because of definitional problems in the *Diagnostic and Statistical Manual of Mental Disorders*, third edition (DSM-III) and the lack of consideration of severity of the anxiety disorder, evidence from animal laboratories (as well as other clinical disorders reviewed below) is more striking (Barlow, 1988). Ancient and seemingly innate defensive reactions, such as freezing when under attack by a predator and fainting at the sight of blood or injections, are highly familial and almost certainly heritable. For example, fully 67% of blood phobics report biological relatives with the same reaction (Ost, Lindahl, Sterner, & Jerremalm, 1984). In addition, panic attacks in nonclinical panickers are strongly familial (Norton, Dorward, & Cox, 1986), despite the fact that little or no anxiety over these attacks is present. Thus, the action tendency of panic may have a distinct genetic component that differs from heritable qualities associated with the trait of anxiety (Eysenck, 1970; Barlow, 1988).

Some evidence exists supporting a similar distinction between endogenous depression on the one hand and exogenous or "neurotic" depression on the other hand. In DSM-III neurotic depression was also termed "major depression without melancholia," and melancholia became one subtype of major depression. Although these distinctions are still problematic (e.g., Akiskal, Bitar, Puzantian, Rosenthal, & Walker, 1978), some evidence suggests that endogenous depression may appear suddenly as if "out of the blue," and may be associated with stronger, healthier premorbid functioning than neurotic depression. Neurotic depression, on the other hand, is thought to be more closely associated with what may be construed as uncontrollable or unpredictable life events or life stressors. Endogenous depression also seems to run more strongly in families and therefore perhaps is associated with stronger biological underpinnings (Zimmerman, Coryell, Pfohl, & Stangl, 1986; Akiskal, 1985). Watson and Kendall (1989) make the case that the primary distinguishing feature of depression, that is, low positive affect manifested by motor retardation and anhedonia, may specifically characterize endogenous depression, "neurotic" depression being less severe and more variable. This analysis suggests that endogenous depression could be considered a phenomenological equivalent of panic, with its "out-of-the-blue" quality, its strong biological underpinnings, and the consistent and severe presentation of low positive affect. The implications of this phenomenological similarity are now pursued.

DISORDERS OF EMOTION: DOUBLE DEPRESSION AND DOUBLE ANXIETY

Elsewhere, I have outlined a model of panic disorder (Barlow, 1988, in press). This model posits that panic attacks seem to occur with some frequency in the normal population, but that panic disorder develops when *anxiety* is focused on the possibility of another "spontaneous" uncontrollable attack occurring. The analyses of anxiety above suggest that the vulnerabilities to become anxious—and most likely the actual presence of generalized anxiety itself, with its characteristic early onset and chronicity (Barlow et al., 1986)—would predate the first panic. But once the panic occurs, it becomes the focus of anxious apprehension.

What is fascinating is that a similar phenomenon seems to occur in depressive disorders. It would be symmetrical for the model if some individuals experience a fundamental basic emotion of sadness/distress in the same way they seem to experience the basic emotion of fear or panic. That is, much as one seems to experience a false alarm, one may feel sadness/distress for no discernible reason (unexpected and uncued), which may then be experienced as unpredictable and/or uncontrollable. The models presented above suggest that the experience of this emotion may be sufficient to trigger anxiety and/or depression in those vulnerable to this affective state. Others without those vulnerabilities may not experience anxiety or depression.

Clinically, this seems to happen. Keller and Shapiro (1982) and others (e.g., Miller, Norman, & Dow, 1986) have described the phenomenon of "double depression," in which bouts of acute and deep depression are superimposed on a preexisting chronic dysthymic state. This is widely observed in clinical practice. But John Teasdale (1985) seems to have captured the essence of this phenomenon most completely when he says,

> It is not uncommon for depressed patients to misinterpret symptoms of depression as signs of irremediable personal inadequacy: for example, the lack of energy, irritability or loss of interest and affection that characterizes depression are seen as signs of selfishness, weakness, or as evidence that a person is a poor wife or mother. Such interpretations, as well as making the symptoms more aversive, imply that they are going to be very difficult to control. (p. 160)

In other words, the experience of the basic emotion of sadness or depression itself is perceived as uncontrollable in these patients. This "psychomotor shutdown" experience, which is perceived as unpredictable and uncontrollable, may be endogenous depression. If we assume for the moment that this is the case, then the term "neurotic depression" seems appropriate to refer to that stage of anxious apprehension in which coping mechanisms are strained and "hopelessness" appears. This term would encompass what Abramson, Metalsky, and Alloy (1989), as well as Alloy, Kelly, Mineka, and Clements (1990), have referred to as "hopelessness depression."

According to this terminology, anxious/neurotically depressed patients may become increasingly hopeless, but very few of them go into a profound psychomotor retardation (with accompanying neurobiological and psychophysiological shutdown and anhedonia) for more than a brief period of time. As noted above, it is also not unusual for these periods of extreme sadness to appear "out of the blue" or for no apparent reason. Finally, these bouts of sadness or major depression can occur outside of the context of a clinical disorder, such as when a loved one dies. The profound sadness with all of the accompanying symptoms are there, but as the grief process ensues, it passes. In addition, Keller and Lavori (1984) observed that 97% of patients they had studied with double depression had recovered from their major depressive episode at a follow-up period. But very few had recovered from their dysthymia (Keller, Lavori, Endicott, Coryell, & Klerman, 1983).

These observations reflect the fact that panic attacks, as well as periods of sadness or "endogenous" depression, are fundamentally self-limiting. In addition, 50% of people who are neurotically depressed (dysthymia, major depression without melancholia) or hopeless experience panic attacks, according to recent evidence from our clinic (Benshoof, 1987). Bouts of endogenous depression may occur across the spectrum of helplessness and hopelessness. This suggests a relative independence of these basic emotions of panic (fear) and endogenous depression (sadness/distress) from the more chronic states of anxiety and dysthymia or dysphoria. This independence may also account for the conflicting and contradictory results emanating from neurobiological studies of anxiety and depression (see Barlow, 1988, and Chapter 3, this volume). Neurotic depression should be essentially similar to anxiety at a neurobiological level, but endogenous depression (low positive affect) should be different.

The origins of the first panic attack or endogenous depressive episode are discussed elsewhere (Barlow, 1988), but suffice it to say that there are marked similarities in their origins. In any case, the central focus of perceptions of uncontrollability (in my view) becomes the unpredictable, unexpected, and uncued negative emotions themselves. I would suggest that this is at the core of emotional disorders, as reflected in Figure 1.5.

Of course, one does not need the very visible and central feature of a panic attack or endogenous depressive episode to present with a severe emotional disorder. Earlier, I have described how chronic and severe anxious apprehension in and of itself can result in substantial disruptions in performance and interference with functioning, even if the focus is rather diffuse. As I have speculated elsewhere (Barlow, 1988), generalized anxiety disorder may be the more chronic and severe disorder in the long run, in that it has an earlier onset, runs a longer course, and seems more difficult to treat than other anxiety disorders, such as panic disorder (which is certainly more problematic for a brief period of time). Akiskal (1983) suggests that dysthymic disorders are also chronic, run a longer course, and can be more difficult to treat than major depressive episodes. Now Daniel Klein and his colleagues (Klein, Taylor, Dickstein, & Harding,

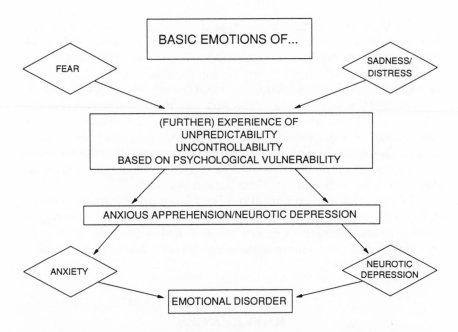

FIGURE 1.5. The relationship of fear (alarm), depression (sadness), anxiety, and dysthymia. Adapted from Barlow, D. H. (1988). *Anxiety and its disorders: The nature and treatment of anxiety and panic* (p. 282). New York: Guilford Press. Copyright 1988 by The Guilford Press. Reprinted with permission.

1988) have demonstrated that clients presenting with primary early-onset dysthymia exhibit greater global impairment, an earlier age of onset of major depression, and a greater likelihood of having recurrent major depressive episodes than a group of clients without dysthymia undergoing a major depressive episode. Interestingly, the dysthymic patients also present with more substantial family histories of affective and antisocial personality disorders and report higher levels of negative stressful life events. This leads Klein et al. to conclude that in the long run, dysthymia is the more severe form of affective disorder.

There is little question that dysthymia—or, to use my preferred term, neurotic depression—subsumes a range of presentations, from subthreshold mood disorders to deeply imbedded traits of character (Akiskal, 1983). Similarly, anxiety can range from a rather mild set of anxious symptoms to a more stable trait (Eysenck, 1970). But what is important is that transitory emotional states of panic or depression can develop an intricate functional relationship with these more chronic affective states.

For this reason, anxious apprehension and neurotic depression, which seem to flow on a continuum and are differentiated most successfully (and perhaps only) by cognitive content (Kendall & Ingram, 1989; see Chapter 8, this volume), are at the heart of emotional disorders. Without this presentation, panic attacks would be "nonclinical" (e.g., Telch, Lucas, & Nelson, 1989) and endogenous depressive episodes would be far less severe (Klein et al., 1988). Although panic attacks and major depressive episodes pass quickly, it is this negative affective state that is chronic and difficult to treat. Only when breakthroughs occur in the understanding and treatment of anxiety/neurotic depression will we unlock the secrets of emotional disorders. It is to this task that this book is devoted.

Of course, not all authors in this book share my theoretical point of view (particularly on the relation of anxiety and depression), but all recognize the severity and chronicity of general anxiety as well as "neurotic" depression, and are striving from various approaches toward a deeper understanding of this affective state.

REFERENCES

Abramson, L. Y., Metalsky, G. I., & Alloy, L. B. (1989). Hopelessness and depression: A theory based subtype of depression. *Psychological Review*, *96*, 358–392.

Akiskal, H. S. (1983). Dysthymic disorder: Psychopathology of proposed chronic depressive subtypes. *American Journal of Psychiatry*, *140*, 11–20.

Akiskal, H. S. (1985). Anxiety: Definition, relationship to depression, and proposal for an integrative model. In A. H. Tuma & J. D. Maser (Eds.), *Anxiety and the anxiety disorders*. Hillside, NJ: Erlbaum.

Akiskal, H. S., Bitar, A. H., Puzantian, V. R., Rosenthal, T. L., & Walker, P. W. (1978). The nosological status of neurotic depression. *Archives of General Psychiatry*, *35*, 756–766.

Alloy, L. B., Kelly, K. A., Mineka, S., & Clements, C. M. (1990). Comorbidity of anxiety and depressive disorders: A helplessness–hopelessness perspective. In J. D. Maser & C. M. Cloninger (Eds.), *Comorbidity of mood and anxiety disorders*. Washington, DC: American Psychiatric Press.

Avery, D. H., Osgood, T. B., Ishiki, D. M., Wilson, L. G., Kenny, M., & Dunnar, D. L. (1985). The DST in psychiatric outpatients with generalized anxiety disorder, panic disorder, or primary affective disorder. *American Journal of Psychiatry*, *142*, 844–848.

Ballenger, J. C., Burrows, G. D., DuPont, R. L., Lesser, I. M., Noyes, R., Pecknold, J. C., Rifkin, A., Swinson, R. P. (1988). Alprazolam in panic disorder and agoraphobia: Results from a multicenter trial. I. Efficacy in short term treatment. *Archives of General Psychiatry*, *45*, 423–428.

Barlow, D. H. (1983, October). *The classification of anxiety disorders*. Paper presented at the conference DSM-III: An Interim Appraisal, sponsored by the American Psychiatric Association, Washington, DC.

Barlow, D. H. (1985). The dimensions of anxiety disorders. In A. H. Tuma & J. D. Maser (Eds.), *Anxiety and the anxiety disorders*. Hillside, NJ: Erlbaum.

Barlow, D. H. (1988). *Anxiety and its disorders: The nature and treatment of anxiety and panic*. New York: Guilford Press.

Barlow, D. H. (in press). Disorders of emotion. *Psychological Inquiry*.

Barlow, D. H., & Craske, M. G. (1990). *"Unexpected" panic and DSM-IV*. Unpublished DSM-IV position paper, American Psychiatric Association, Washington, DC.

Barlow, D. H., Di Nardo, P. A., Vermilyea, B. B., Vermilyea, J. A., & Blanchard, E. B. (1986). Co-morbidity and depression among the anxiety disorders: Issues in diagnosis and classification. *Journal of Nervous and Mental Disease*, *174*, 63–72.

Barlow, D. H., Vermilyea, J., Blanchard, E. B., Vermilyea, B. B., Di Nardo, P. A., & Cerny, J. A. (1985). The phenomenon of panic. *Journal of Abnormal Psychology*, *94*, 320–328.

Beck, A. T., Emery, G., & Greenberg, R. (1985). *Anxiety disorders and phobias: A cognitive perspective*. New York: Basic Books.

Benshoof, B. G. (1987). *A comparison of anxiety and depressive symptomatology in the anxiety and affective disorders*. Unpublished doctoral dissertation, State University of New York at Albany.

Breier, A., Charney, D. S., & Heninger, G. R. (1985). The diagnostic validity of anxiety disorders and their relationship to depressive illness. *American Journal of Psychiatry*, *142*, 787–797.

Cannon, W. B. (1929). *Bodily changes in pain, hunger, fear and rage* (2nd ed.). New York: Appleton-Century & Crofts.

Carver, C. S., & Scheier, M. F. (1981). *Attention and self-regulation: A control theory approach to human behavior*. New York: Springer-Verlag.

Cloninger, C. R. (1986). A unified biosocial theory of personality and its role in the development of anxiety states. *Psychiatric Development*, *3*, 167–226.

Cohen, A. S., Barlow, D. H., & Blanchard, E. B. (1985). The psychophysiology of relaxation associated panic attacks. *Journal of Abnormal Psychology*, *94*, 96–101.

Coryell, W., Noyes, R., Clancy, J., Crowe, R., & Chaudhry, D. (1985). Abnormal escape from dexamethasome suppression in agoraphobia with panic attacks. *Psychiatry Research*, *15*, 301–311.

Darwin, C. R. (1872). *The expression of emotions in man and animals*. London: John Murray.

Di Nardo, P. A., & Barlow, D. H. (1990). Syndrome and symptom co-occurrence in the anxiety disorders. In J. D. Maser & C. R. Cloninger (Eds.), *Comorbidity of mood and anxiety disorders*. Washington, DC: American Psychiatric Press.

Dobson, K. S. (1985). The relationship between anxiety and depression. *Clinical Psychology Review*, *5*, 307–324.

Eysenck, H. J. (Ed.). (1967). *The biological basis of personality*. Springfield, IL: Charles C Thomas.

Eysenck, H. J. (1970). *The structure of human personality*. London: Methuen.

Eysenck, H. J. (Ed.). (1981). *A model for personality*. New York: Springer-Verlag.

Fridlund, A. J., Hatfield, M. E., Cottam, G. L., & Fowler, J. C. (1986). Anxiety and striate-muscle activation: Evidence from electromyographic pattern analysis. *Journal of Abnormal Psychology, 95*, 228–236.

Gotlieb, I. H. (1984). Depression and general psychopathology in university students. *Journal of Abnormal Psychology, 93*, 19–30.

Gotlieb, I. H., & Cane, D. B. (1989). Self-report assessment of depression and anxiety. In P. C. Kendall & D. Watson (Eds.), *Anxiety and depression: Distinctive and overlapping features*. San Diego: Academic Press.

Gray, J. A. (1982). *The neuropsychology of anxiety*. New York: Oxford University Press.

Gray, J. A. (1985). Issues in the neuropsychology of anxiety. In A. H. Tuma & J. D. Maser (Eds.), *Anxiety and the anxiety disorders*. Hillsdale, NJ: Erlbaum.

Hamilton, M. (1959). The assessment of anxiety states by rating. *British Journal of Medical Psychology, 32*, 50–55.

Hamilton, M. (1960). A rating scale for depression. *Journal of Neurology, Neurosurgery and Psychiatry, 23*, 56–62.

Heimberg, R. G., Vermilyea, J. A., Dodge, C. S., Becker, R. E., & Barlow, D. H. (1987). Attributional style, depression, and anxiety: An evaluation of the specificity of depressive attributions. *Cognitive Therapy and Research, 11*, 537–550.

Izard, C. E. (Ed.). (1977). *Human emotions*. New York: Plenum Press.

Izard, C. E., & Blumberg, M. A. (1985). Emotion theory and the role of emotions in anxiety in children and adults. In A. H. Tuma & J. D. Maser (Eds.), *Anxiety and the anxiety disorders*. Hillsdale, NJ: Erlbaum.

Kahn, J. P., Stevenson, E., Topol, P., & Klein, D. (1986). Agitated depression, alprazolam, and panic anxiety. *American Journal of Psychiatry, 143*, 1172–1173.

Keller, M. B., & Lavori, P. W. (1984). Double depression, major depression and dysthymia: Distinct entities or different phases of a single disorder? *Psychopharmacology Bulletin, 20*, 399–402.

Keller, M. B., Lavori, P. W., Endicott, J., Coryell, W., & Klerman, G. L. (1983). "Double depression": Two-year follow-up. *American Journal of Psychiatry, 140*, 689–694.

Keller, M. B., & Shapiro, R. W. (1982). "Double depression": Superimposition of acute depressive episodes on chronic depressive disorders. *American Journal of Psychiatry, 139*, 438–442.

Kendall, P. C., & Ingram, R. I. (1989). Cognitive–behavioral perspectives: Theory and research on depression and anxiety. In P. C. Kendall & D. Watson (Eds.), *Anxiety and depression: Distinctive and overlapping features*. San Diego: Academic Press.

Kendall, P. C., & Watson, D. (Eds.). (1989). *Anxiety and depression: Distinctive and overlapping features.* San Diego: Academic Press.

Klein, D. F., Rabkin, J. G., & Gorman, J. M. (1985). Etiological and pathophysiological inferences from the pharmacological treatment of anxiety. In A. H. Tuma & J. D. Maser (Eds.), *Anxiety and the anxiety disorders.* Hillsdale, NJ: Erlbaum.

Klein, D. N., Taylor, E. B., Dickstein, S., & Harding, K. (1988). Primary early-onset dysthymia: Comparison with primary nonbipolar nonchronic major depression on demographic, clinical, familial, personality, and socioenvironmental characteristics and short-term outcome. *Journal of Abnormal Psychology, 97*, 387–398.

Korchin, S. (1964). Anxiety and cognition. In C. Scheerer (Ed.), *Cognition: Theory, research, and practice.* New York: Harper & Row.

Lang, P. J. (1979). A bio-informational theory of emotional imagery. *Psychophysiology, 16*, 495–512.

Lang, P. J. (1984). Cognition in emotion: Concept and action. In C. Izard, J. Kagan, & R. B. Zajonc (Eds.), *Emotion, cognition and behavior.* New York: Cambridge University Press.

Lang, P. J. (1985). The cognitive psychophysiology of emotion: Fear and anxiety. In A. H. Tuma & J. D. Maser (Eds.), *Anxiety and the anxiety disorders.* Hillsdale, NJ: Erlbaum.

Lazarus, R. S. (1968). Emotions and adaptation: Conceptual and empirical relations. In W. J. Arnold (Ed.), *Nebraska Symposium on Motivation* (Vol. 16). Lincoln: University of Nebraska Press.

Leckman, J. F., Weissman, M. M., Merikangas, K. R., Pauls, D. L., & Prusoff, B. A. (1983). Panic disorder and major depression. *Archives of General Psychiatry, 40*, 1055–1060.

Liddell, H. S. (1949). The role of vigilance in the development of animal neurosis. In P. Hoch & J. Zubin (Eds.), *Anxiety.* New York: Grune & Stratton.

MacLeod, C., Mathews, A., & Tata, P. (1986). Attentional bias in emotional disorders. *Journal of Abnormal Psychology, 95*, 15–20.

Mandler, G. (1966). Anxiety. In D. L. Sills (Ed.), *International encyclopedia of the social sciences.* New York: Macmillan.

Mavissakalian, M. (1987). Initial depression and response to imipramine in agoraphobia. *Journal of Nervous and Mental Disease, 175*, 358–361.

Mavissakalian, M., & Michelson, L. (1986). Agoraphobia: Relative and combined effectiveness of therapist-assisted *in vivo* exposure and imipramine. *Journal of Clinical Psychiatry, 47*, 117–122.

McCauley, P. A., Di Nardo, P. A., & Barlow, D. H. (1987, November). *Differentiating anxiety and depression using a modified scoring system for the Hamilton scales.* Poster presented at the annual meeting of the Association for Advancement of Behavior Therapy, Boston.

Miller, I. W., Norman, W. H., & Dow, M. G. (1986). Psychosocial characteristics of "double depression." *American Journal of Psychiatry, 143*, 1042–1044.

Mineka, S. (1985a). Animal models of anxiety-based disorders: Their usefulness and limitations. In A. H. Tuma & J. D. Maser (Eds.), *Anxiety and the anxiety disorders*. Hillsdale, NJ: Erlbaum.

Mineka, S. (1985b). The frightful complexity of the origins of fears. In Bruch & J. B. Overmier (Eds.), *Affect, conditioning, and cognition: Essays on the determinants of behavior*. Hillside, NJ: Erlbaum.

Mineka, S., Gunnar, M., & Champoux, M. (1986). Control and early socioemotional development: Infant rhesus monkeys reared in controllable versus uncontrollable environments. *Child Development, 57*, 1241–1256.

Mineka, S., & Kihlstrom, J. (1978). Unpredictable and uncontrollable aversive events. *Journal of Abnormal Psychology, 87*, 256–271.

Norton, R. G., Dorward, J., & Cox, B. J. (1986). Factors associated with panic attacks in nonclinical subjects. *Behavior Therapy, 17*, 239–252.

Ost, L. G., Lindahl, I. L., Sterner, U., & Jerremalm, A. (1984). Exposure *in vivo* vs. applied relaxation in the treatment of blood phobia. *Behaviour Research and Therapy, 22*, 205–216.

Peterson, C., Semmel, A., von Baeyer, C., Abramson, L. Y., Metalsky, G. I., & Seligman, M. E. P. (1982). The Attributional Style Questionnaire. *Cognitive Therapy and Research, 6*, 287–299.

Puig-Antich, J., & Rabinovich, H. (1986). Relationship between affective and anxiety disorders in childhood. In R. G. Helman (Ed.), *Anxiety disorders of childhood*. New York: Wiley.

Rachman, S., & Levitt, K. (1985). Panics and their consequences. *Behaviour Research and Therapy, 23*, 585–600.

Rapee, R. (1985). A distinction between panic disorder and generalized anxiety disorder: Clinical presentation. *Australian and New Zealand Journal of Psychiatry, 19*, 227–232.

Rickels, K., Feighner, J. P., & Smith, W. T. (1985). Alprazolam and amitriptyline, doxepin and placebo in the treatment of depression. *Archives of General Psychiatry, 42*, 134–141.

Riskind, J. H., Beck, A. T., Brown, G., & Steer, R. A. (1987). Taking the measure of anxiety and depression: Validity of the reconstructed Hamilton scales. *Journal of Nervous and Mental Disease, 175*, 474–479.

Roth, M., Gurney, C., Garside, R. F., & Kerr, T. A. (1972). Studies in the classification of affective disorders: Relationship between anxiety states and depressive illness—I. *British Journal of Psychiatry, 121*, 147–161.

Rotter, J. B. (1954). *Social learning and clinical psychology*. Englewood Cliffs, NJ: Prentice-Hall.

Roy-Byrne, P. P., Bierer, L. M., & Uhde, T. W. (1985). The dexamethasone suppression test in panic disorder: Comparison with normal controls. *Biological Psychiatry, 20*, 1237–1240.

Roy-Byrne, P. P., Mellman, T. A., & Uhde, T. W. (1988). Biologic findings in panic disorder: Neuroendocrine and sleep-related abnormalities. *Journal of Anxiety Disorders, 2*, 17–29.

Sanderson, W. C., Di Nardo, P. A., Rapee, R. M., & Barlow, D. H. (1990). Syndrome co-morbidity in patients diagnosed with a DSM-III-Revised anxiety disorder. *Journal of Abnormal Psychology, 99*, 308–312.

Sartory, G. (1986). Effect of phobic anxiety on the orienting response. *Behaviour Research and Therapy, 24*, 251–261.

Scheier, M. F., Carver, C. S., & Matthews, K. A. (1983). Attentional factors in the perception of bodily states. In J. T. Cacioppo & R. E. Petty (Eds.), *Social psychophysiology: A source book*. New York: Guilford Press.

Schwartz, G. E. (1976). Self-regulation of response patterning: Implications for psychophysiological research and therapy. *Biofeedback and Self-Regulation, 1*, 7–30.

Schweizer, E. E., Swenson, C. M., Winokur, A., Rickels, K., & Maislin, G. (1986). The dexamethasone suppression test in generalized anxiety disorder. *British Journal of Psychiatry, 149*, 320–322.

Seligman, M. E. P. (1975). *Helplessness*. San Francisco: W. H. Freeman.

Shapiro, D. (1974). Operant-feedback control of human blood pressure: Some clinical issues. In P. A. Obrist, A. H. Black, J. Brener, & L. V. DiCara (Eds.), *Cardiovascular psychophysiology: Current issues in response mechanisms, biofeedback and methodology*. Chicago: Aldine.

Spielberger, C. D., Gorsuch, R. L., & Lushene, R. E. (1970). *Manual for the State–Trait Anxiety Inventory*. Palo Alto, CA: Consulting Psychologists Press.

Spielberger, C. D. (1985). Anxiety, cognition, and affect: A state-trait perspective. In A. H. Tuma & J. D. Maser (Eds.), *Anxiety and the anxiety disorders*. Hillsdale, NJ: Erlbaum.

Taylor, C. B., Sheikh, J., Agras, W. S., Roth, W. T., Margraf, J., Ehlers, A., Maddock, R. J., & Gossard, D. (1986). Self-report of panic attacks: Agreement with heart rate changes. *American Journal of Psychiatry, 143*, 478–482.

Teasdale, J. D. (1985). Psychological treatments for depression: How do they work? *Behaviour Research and Therapy, 23*, 157–165.

Telch, M. J., Lucas, J. A., & Nelson, P. (1989). Nonclinical panic in college students: An investigation of prevalence and symptomatology. *Journal of Abnormal Psychology, 98*, 300–306.

Tellegen, A. (1985). Structures of mood and personality and their relevance to assessing anxiety, with an emphasis on self-report. In A. H. Tuma & J. D. Maser (Eds.), *Anxiety and the anxiety disorders*. Hillsdale, NJ: Erlbaum.

Watson, D., Clark, L. A., & Carey, G. (1988). Positive and negative affectivity and their relation to anxiety and depressive disorders. *Journal of Abnormal Psychology, 97*, 346–353.

Watson, D., & Kendall, P. C. (1989). Understanding anxiety and depression: Their relation to negative and positive affective states. In P. C. Kendall & D. Watson (Eds.), *Anxiety and depression: Distinctive and overlapping features*. San Diego: Academic Press.

Weissman, M. M. (1985). The epidemiology of anxiety disorders: Rates, risks and familial patterns. In A. H. Tuma & J. D. Maser (Eds.), *Anxiety and the anxiety disorders*. Hillsdale, NJ: Erlbaum.

Yerkes, R. M., & Dobson, J. D. (1908). The relation of strength of stimulus to rapidity of habit-formation. *Journal of Comparative Neurology and Psychology, 18*, 459–482.

Zillmann, D. (1983). Arousal and aggression. In R. G. Geen & E. Donnerstein (Eds.), *Aggression: Theoretical and empirical reviews* (Vol. 1). New York: Academic Press.

Zimmerman, M., Coryell, W., Pfohl, B., & Stangl, D. (1986). The validity of four concepts of endogenous depression. *Archives of General Psychiatry, 43,* 111–122.

Zung, W. W. (1965). A self-rating depression scale. *Archives of General Psychiatry, 12,* 63–70.

2

The Nature of Normal and Pathological Worry

THOMAS D. BORKOVEC
RICHARD N. SHADICK
MILDRED HOPKINS
Penn State University

Our topic in this chapter is the nature of normal and pathological worry. Excessive and/or unrealistic worry about two or more life circumstances unrelated to other Axis I disorders is the central diagnostic feature of generalized anxiety disorder (GAD) in the *Diagnostic and Statistical Manual of Mental Disorders*, third edition, revised (DSM-III-R) (see Chapter 5), although worry is also present in several other disorders. The topic thus partly relates to such diagnostic issues as the threshold at which normal worry becomes diagnosable as GAD, the definition of the terms "excessive" and "unrealistic," and the specification of spheres of worry content distinctive of GAD and other disorders. However, it also partly relates to more fundamental questions about the similarities or differences in worry between normal and clinical groups, as well as the functions that the worry process may have in the maintenance of anxiety disorders. Unfortunately, little research on worry exists among clinical samples, making it difficult to draw firm conclusions about some of these questions. Consequently, one of the goals of our review is the identification of fruitful areas for further exploration to address these questions, based on a summary of what is currently known about the nature of worry in normal samples and the small amount of investigation on clinical (largely GAD) samples. Thus, the main review sections end with conclusions relevant to such future research. The second major goal of the chapter is to present a theoretical model of the nature and functions of worry. Hints from the extant literature suggest that (1) worry may be negatively reinforced by somatic anxiety reduction, and (2) the worry process may itself preclude emotional processing in such a way that emotional change is prevented and anxiety is maintained.

REVIEW OF WORRY RESEARCH

From our review, three common themes emerge from both the normal and clinical literature on worry. First, both areas have produced some data bearing on the spheres, or content domains, of worry. Second, each area has measured certain salient dimensions of worry-like phenomena (e.g., cognitive intrusions), such as frequency, intensity, uncontrollability, and disruptiveness. Third, both research areas have assessed the relationship of worry or cognitive intrusion to the somatic aspects of anxiety. Because this relationship bears on the nature of worry, and because diagnosis of GAD and other anxiety disorders also requires the presence of some somatic symptoms, we feel that a review of recent studies addressing this relationship is relevant. The reviews of recent research on both normal worry and clinical worry are organized around these three themes.

Studies on Normal Samples

Spheres of Worry

Four investigations have asked normal samples to rate the degree to which certain *a priori* topics were worrisome to them. Among children, the family was found to be the topic of most frequent concern (and animals and finances the least) for the total group (n = 854) in two studies (Simon & Ward, 1974, 1982). Significant gender effects indicated in one study that girls worried more about family-related, social, school-related, and imagination topics, and that older children had significantly fewer worries. Teacher rankings of a subset of 60 children for degree of worry correlated quite highly with the children's total worry scores. In a group of 74 college students, academic and interpersonal worries were rated as most frequent, whereas concerns about physical harm were least frequent (Borkovec, Robinson, Pruzinsky, & DePree, 1983). No differences were found between self-labeled "worriers" and "nonworriers" on these topic frequencies except by gender: Male worriers were more often concerned with interpersonal issues than were male nonworriers, whereas female worriers more frequently worried about financial and academic topics than did female nonworriers. Among elderly subjects (n = 121), health concerns were the most highly rated, followed by social relations and finances (Wisocki, 1988). Neither gender nor marital status was related to these ratings, although increasing age understandably correlated significantly with worries about health, and preretirement income correlated with worries about finances.

Dimensions of Worry and Intrusive Thoughts

Considerable research has been conducted on certain dimensionalized characteristics of intrusive thinking among normal subjects. In summary, negative intrusive thoughts are typified by reports of greater frequency, intensity, disruption, uncontrollability, and unpleasantness than are neutral thoughts. Both traits and state conditions have been shown to contribute to these parameters. Emerging from this literature is the conclusion that, although cause–effect relationships have yet to be determined among dimensions, uncontrollability (or the difficulty of dismissal) seems to be the most central feature of worry and intrusive thinking. This dimension is found to be significantly correlated most frequently with the other assessed dimensions (Salkovskis & Harrison, 1984), and most often is affected by dispositional group comparisons or experimental manipulations, as exemplified below.

Uncontrollability of negative thinking correlates with intensity and frequency of such thoughts in numerous studies (Clark, 1986; Clark & DeSilva, 1985; England & Dickerson, 1988; Kent & Jambunathan, 1989; Parkinson & Rachman, 1981; Salkovskis & Harrison, 1984). Induced intrusive thoughts (Edwards & Dickerson, 1987a; Sutherland, Newman, & Rachman, 1982), as well as naturally occurring intrusions of high frequency (Parkinson & Rachman, 1981), are harder to dismiss than neutral thoughts or low-frequency intrusions; moreover, the amount of worry associated with the thought correlates with its uncontrollability to a greater degree than the subjective tension induced by the thought (Clark, 1986). In a longitudinal study (Kent & Jambunathan, 1989), medical students who increased in state anxiety over a 4- to 5-week period approaching final exams also reported increased uncontrollability, distress, and frequency of intrusive thoughts. These thoughts became increasingly negative in content, relative to the thoughts of students showing no change or declines in state anxiety. Regression analysis revealed uncontrollability to account for the greatest amount of variance in anxiety change. These findings occurred despite the fact that no differences were found in subjective probability of negative outcomes over time or between groups. Although intrusive thoughts that are anxiety-provoking and those that are depressing share some features (Clark & De Silva, 1985), the former are more difficult to dismiss (Clark, 1986), and sad mood tends to increase this uncontrollability (Edwards & Dickerson, 1987b; Sutherland et al., 1982). Intrusive thoughts are harder to dismiss than are intrusive images, even though the latter are rated as more unacceptable (Parkinson & Rachman, 1981). Traits of anxiety (Eysenck, 1984), chronic worry (Borkovec et al., 1983), and intrusive-thought style (Clark, 1986; Sarason, Sarason, Keefe, Hayes, & Shearin, 1986) predict greater uncontrollability of negative intrusive thoughts in the laboratory. Intrusive-thought style as a trait predicts more rapid formation of negative thoughts (Clark, 1986), although speed of formation does not distinguish neutral- or intrusive-thought generation in unselected samples (Sutherland et al., 1982). Induction of an anxious state stimulates the initiation of intrusive thought, whereas trait anxiety contributes to its maintenance (Eysenck, 1984). Worriers report greater worrying during relaxation than during baseline, as well as in comparison to nonworriers (Carter, Johnson, & Borkovec, 1986). Worriers have greater difficulty concentrating attention on a task or making decisions and dismissing intruding negative thoughts than do nonworriers, whereas all subjects (regardless of trait status) show an increased inability to dismiss such thoughts and to concentrate or make decisions after an "incubating" state period of worrying about a topic of current concern (Borkovec et al., 1983; Metzger, Miller, Cohen, Sofka, & Borkevec, 1990; York, Borkovec, Vasey, & Stern, 1987). Thus, worry has significant effects on attentional and decision-making processes.

Relationship of Worry to Somatic Aspects of Anxiety

Several investigations have documented that worry is a component of anxiety, separate from its somatic aspects and cognitive in nature. Two decades of text anxiety research have revealed (1) the partial independence of worry and perceived sensations of somatic anxiety, and (2) the greater power of worry than of somatic measures for predicting test-related per-formance (e.g., Deffenbacher, 1977, 1986; Morris, Davis, & Hutchings, 1981). Worry has been found to correlate more highly than tension reports with other measures of emotional disturbance, such as the State–Trait Anxiety Inventory Trait scale, the Beck Depression Inventory, and numerous fear survey items, especially those having to having to do with social evaluation (Borkovec et al., 1983). This social-evaluative quality of worry may relate to the high frequency of social phobia as a secondary diagnosis among GAD clients (Sanderson & Barlow, 1990; see also Chapter 6). Degree of difficulty in dismissing intrusive negative thoughts also correlates more highly with degree of worrisome experience than with amount of reported general tension (Clark, 1986). High degrees of worry among civilians exposed to war are related to variable degrees of "fear" report, and low levels of "fear" are associated with variable degrees of worry (Levy & Guttman, 1976). Somatic symptoms during worry are reported to be only of relatively modest intensity, with muscle tension and upset stomach being most often indicated (Borkevec et al., 1983; Hatfield, Doyle, & Borkovec, 1981). Induction of worry produces a greater increase in negative cognitive intrusions during a subsequent attention-focusing task than neutral induction, whereas somatic anxiety induction does not (York et al., 1987).

Worry also does not produce much peripheral physiological activation (Deffenbacher, 1980; Karteroliotis & Gill, 1987). Differences have not been generally found between self-labeled worriers and nonworriers during rest or during worry periods when subjects are asked to worry in their customary fashion (Borkovec et al., 1983; McCarthy & Borkovec, 1983). Nor has degree of controllability of intrusive thoughts correlated with multiple physiological measures (Clark, 1986). Interestingly, thoughts (reported by 96.8% of normals having intrusive activity) have been found to predominate over images (reported by 66.7%) in intrusive cognition (Parkinson & Rachman, 1981)—a finding replicated in a clinical GAD sample to be discussed later. Given the general absence of autonomic changes due to worry, and the predominance of thought over images in cognitive intrusions, it is of significance that central physiological events have been found to mark the occurrence of worry: Worriers and nonworriers both show a significant increase in electroencephalographic (EEG) beta activity in the frontal lobes when instructed to worry, and worriers show a greater shift toward left, as opposed to right, frontal activation (Carter et al., 1986).

Conclusions

1. The frequency of content domains tends to vary with subjects' general current life conditions. In the only study to contrast self-labeled worriers and nonworriers, no differences were found in the significance of any sphere except by gender.

2. In normal worry, the process is predominantly cognitive in nature; is associated with little perceived or actual peripheral physiological activation; and correlates more often with performance disruption, other measures of emotional disturbance (especially social-evaluative anxieties), difficulty of dismissal of negative thoughts, and increased subsequent intrusions of negative thoughts than does somatic anxiety.

3. Although worry and intrusive thoughts are characterized by high frequency, intensity, and disruption of attention and decision making, uncontrollability may be their most salient feature.

4. Both state (sad mood, anxiety induction, worry induction, relaxation) and trait (trait anxiety, self-labeled worry status, intrusive-thought style) variables influence the uncontrollability, frequency, intensity, and disrup-

tiveness of negative thoughts. Subjects high in trait anxiety are bothered by these thoughts and their dimensions over many environmental conditions, whereas experimental conditions inducing negative states often raise subjects low in trait anxiety to high trait levels. Thus far in several studies, virtually every aspect of worry feature found in highly worried or highly anxious normals has been briefly reproduced in nonanxious normals via an anxiety or worry induction. The only exception has been hemispheric laterality of frontal EEG beta activity.

Studies on Clinical Samples

Spheres of Worry

Table 2.1 presents worry spheres from three investigations of GAD clients. In one study (Sanderson & Barlow, 1990), 14 female and 8 male GAD clients (average age, 43 years; range, 31–63) were identified by DSM-III-R criteria, using the revised version of the Anxiety Disorders Interview Schedule (ADIS-R; Di Nardo & Barlow, 1988). During the interview, clients were asked to provide the content of their worries, which the interviewers classified into one of four general categories. For reliability estimation, 14 of the 22 clients were independently interviewed by a second assessor. Thirty-five specific worries for the 14 clients were identified by the assessors. Interviewers showed an agreement level of 78.6% on content classification. The most common worry category was family; illness was the least frequent concern.

Craske, Rapee, Jackel, and Barlow (1989) replicated aspects of the Sanderson and Barlow (1990) study with a new sample of 19 GAD clients diagnosed with the ADIS-R, and a control group composed of 26 friends of anxiety center clients who had never received treatment for psychological problems. During a 3-week interval, subjects completed a questionnaire on worry content and rating scales regarding their worries as soon as they detected worrying. They did this three consecutive times when they noticed worrying "significantly" or "definitely," as long as those worries were not related to panic attacks or phobias. Content classification on reported worries by two independent judges employed a set of categories similar to that used by Sanderson and Barlow (1990); a "miscellaneous" category was added, however. Independent raters agreed on category assignment in 82% of the 44 resulting GAD worries and 74% of the 62 control worries. For GAD clients, illness/health/injury was the most common category, miscellaneous worries were quite frequent, and finances were of least concern. Controls showed a different ordering, with work/school being the sphere of greatest worry. The two groups differed significantly,

TABLE 2.1. Rank-Ordered Spheres of Worry among GAD Clients and Nonanxious Control Subjects

Sanderson & Barlow (1990)	Craske et al. (1989)		Penn State Project
GAD worries from ADIS-R	*GAD worries* from self-monitoring	*GAD worries* from ADIS-R	*GAD worries* from ADIS-R
Family (79%)	Illness/health/injury (30.6%)	Family/home/ interpersonal (32.2%)	Family/home/ interpersonal (31.3%)
Financial (50%)	Family (27.8%)	Miscellaneous (22.6%)	Miscellaneous (31.3%)
Work (43%)	Miscellaneous (25.2%)	Illness/health/ injury (19.4%)	Work/school (25.4%)
Illness (14%)	Work/school (13.9%)	Work/school (16.1%)	Financial (8.9%)
	Financial (2.8%)	Financial (9.7%)	Illness/health/ injury (3.0%)
	Control worries from self-monitoring		*Control worries* from ADIS-R
	Work/school (30.4%)		Family/home/ interpersonal (43.7%)
	Family/home/ interpersonal (26.1%)		Illness/home/ injury (25%)
	Financial (26.1%)		Work/school (18.7%)
	Miscellaneous (15.2%)		Financial (12.5%)
	Illness/health/injury (2.2%)		Miscellaneous (0%)

Note. Percentages listed for the Sanderson & Barlow (1990) study reflect the number of clients reporting a worry in each sphere; percentages in the other studies reflect the number of specific worries classified in each sphere.

with greater illness concerns among GAD clients and greater financial worries among controls. Two independent judges also categorized worry content from the ADIS-R interview, as in the Sanderson and Barlow (1990) study; interjudged agreement was 91.2% on the 68 worries identified. Percentages in each content area of the judges' classifications were similar to those obtained from the self-monitoring data, except for the illness category.

Although the two groups did not differ significantly on demographic variables in the Craske et al. (1989) study, sufficient variation existed to warrant caution in interpreting the comparisons. The 8 male and 11 female GAD clients tended to be older than the 12 male and 14 female controls (average age 41 vs. 33.5 years), and had a tendency toward higher income and lower education levels. The latter might partially explain the greater concern of controls over financial issues and lesser concern over illness, health, and injury.

The Penn State GAD Project, in its current therapy trial, has accumulated some data relevant to the content classification of worries. During the administration of the ADIS-R by a psychiatric assessor, GAD clients provided 162 topics about which they were currently worried. Sixteen of the clients were female and 15 were male; they averaged 34.1 years in age (range, 17–67). Two independent judges classified the worries into the five spheres used by the Albany project. The miscellaneous category was further subdivided into subcategories currently being employed at Albany (self-worth, daily activities, the future, a miscellaneous subcategory, and "everything"), plus one category regarding environmental issues. The percentage of agreement on the five main categories (82.7%) was very close to that reported by Sanderson and Barlow (1990). After classification of the reliable items, the family/interpersonal and miscellaneous categories contained the most worries, and illness/health/injury the fewest. Agreement on the subcategories of the miscellaneous category was considerably lower (64.3%). Among the 27 reliable items in that category, the greatest number of mentioned worries fell into the topic of self-worth (29.6%), followed by "everything" (18.5%), the miscellaneous subcategory (18.5%), and daily activities, the future, and the environment (11.1% each).

A group of nonanxious subjects, screened via the ADIS-R and matched to the first 13 GAD clients on age, education, gender, and race, also provided worry topics. In contrast to the number of worries reported by the GAD clients (mean = 5.2 per client), controls mentioned very few (mean = 1.23). The independent judges agreed on content classification in 16 of the 17 worries (94.1%). Family/interpersonal was the most common topic area; the miscellaneous category had no representation.

Dimensions of Worry

In addition to content classification of spheres of worry, Sanderson and Barlow (1990) obtained other information relevant to worry in GAD. First, the kappa coefficient of agreement between the two interviewers on whether each of the 35 identified worriers was "excessive and/or unrealistic" was .90. Second, 20 of the 22 clients answered "yes" to whether they worried excessively about minor things, in contrast to the lower rates among other anxiety disorder groups diagnosed by the ADIS-R at the

Albany Center for Stress and Anxiety Disorders. The conditional probability of having a GAD diagnosis, given "yes" to this question, was .36; the probability of not receiving that diagnosis, given "no," was .96. Finally, 19 of the 22 GAD clients reported feeling tense, anxious, or worried for 50% or more of a typical day; two others fell in the 40–49% range; and the last client was in the 20–29% range.

Craske et al. (1989) found the percentage of a typical day spent feeling tense, anxious, or worried during the past month on the ADIS-R to be similar to that reported in the previous study, and significantly greater for GAD clients than for controls. They also had the clients and control subjects rate their self-monitored worries on a variety of dimensional scales. Recognizable precipitants to the initiation of worry were identified by GAD clients (64%) significantly less often than the controls (88%). Interestingly, in normal subjects experiencing frequent intrusive thoughts, a remarkably similar level of precipitant identification (68%) was found (Parkinson & Rachman, 1981). On three additional rating scales in the Craske et al. (1989) study, GAD clients significantly differed from controls: Their worries were less controllable, less realistic, and less successfully reduced by corrective actions. The two groups did not differ on maximum anxiety or aversiveness associated with the worries, likelihood of occurrence of the concerned event, anxiety felt while resisting the worry, or the duration of the worry. In regression analysis, only the controllability rating significantly predicted group membership ($R^2 = .34$).

In the Penn State Project, of 47 clients having a principal diagnosis of GAD, 44 said "yes" to the question, "Do you worry excessively about minor things?" on the ADIS-R. Among clients receiving a secondary diagnosis of GAD, 11 of 14 also answered affirmatively. For those ultimately receiving a different principal anxiety disorder diagnosis without a secondary GAD diagnosis, 12 answered affirmatively, and 5 negatively. In contrast, the nonanxious control group of 13 subjects all answered this question negatively. It was also discovered, however, that there was some degree of unreliability in the answers to this question. Of 25 test–retest reliability checks from dual ADIS-R interviews, clients gave the same answer to different interviewers on 20 of the occasions (80%).

Our ADIS-R interviewers also asked clients to talk about the extent to which their tension, anxiety, and worry interfered with daily functioning, and rated this interference on a 5-point scale. A group of 38 DSM-III-R GAD clients was found to have significantly higher ratings than a group of 8 clients who by initial telephone screening appeared to experience GAD symptoms but were found on subsequent ADIS-R to have another anxiety disorder diagnosis without a secondary GAD diagnosis, $t(45) = 2.68$, $p < .02$. The average rating for GAD clients (2.6) fell between "moderate" and "severe" on the assessor rating scale, whereas that for clients with other anxiety disorders fell between "mild" and "moderate" (1.85).

Assessor ratings of the four DSM-III GAD areas of psychic and somatic symptoms did not distinguish among the various anxiety disorders or major depression in one study (Barlow, Blanchard, Vermilyea, Vermilyea, & Di Nardo, 1986); these symptoms were pervasive throughout and not significantly characteristic of GAD. However, cell sizes were quite small for some of the diagnostic groups. A more recent study indicated that significant differentiation of anxiety groups was possible, using the 13 symptoms clusters from the Hamilton Anxiety Rating Scale (Gross, Oei, & Evans, 1989). Clients (n = 417) who received a diagnosis of GAD, panic disorder, agoraphobia, or social phobia by DSM-III criteria via an unspecified structured interview were also given the Hamilton scale. Discriminant-function analysis indicated that GAD clients scored significantly higher on anxious mood (including worry and anticipation of the worst) than social phobics and panic disorder clients. Agoraphobics fell nonsignificantly between the groups, but scored signficantly higher on items related to fear than the other three groups. Social phobias scored higher than panic disorder clients on autonomic symptoms. Remaining clusters failed to distinguish the groups clearly.

Relationship of Worry to Somatic Aspects of Anxiety

The current DSM-III-R diagnosis of GAD requires the presence of worry, plus some symptoms from the DSM-III areas of vigilance and scanning, motor tension, and autonomic hyperactivity. Although assessor ratings of somatic symptoms have not been found in the main to differentiate significantly among DSM-III anxiety disorders (Barlow et al., 1986; Gross et al., 1989), additional research suggests some somatic differences, both perceived and actual, between GAD and other anxiety groups. In terms of *perceived* sensations, panic disorder clients reported higher somatic symptoms on the Cognitive and Somatic Anxiety Questionnaire than DSM-III-R GAD clients (Di Nardo & Barlow, 1990), although they were equivalent on its cognitive anxiety items. DSM-III-R panic clients have reported that induced hyperventilation symptoms were more like their naturally occurring anxiety symptoms than did GAD clients (Rapee, 1986), and clients with DSM-III panic disorder and agoraphobia with panic disorder have reported higher anxiety and hyperventilation symptoms after a hyperventilation challenge than did a combined group of clients with GAD and social phobia (Holt & Andrews, 1989). Such diagnostic groups differences have not always been replicated, however (de Ruiter, Garssen,

Rijken, & Kraaimaat, 1989). Interestingly, imipramine has a significantly greater effect on psychic symptoms (including negative anticipatory thinking) with DSM-III-R GAD clients, whereas alprazolam has a greater effect on somatic symptoms, suggesting the separateness of these symptom groups (Hoehn-Saric, McLeod, & Zimmerli, 1988a). Morever, the relationship between perceived and actual physiological response is not strong. Although DSM-III-R GAD clients can detect changes in response to stress, they are inaccurate with regard to degree of change (McLeod, Hoehn-Saric, & Stefan, 1986).

A review (Hoehn-Saric & McLeod, 1988) of studies involving physiological monitoring suggests that actual autonomic nervous system activity in GAD clients reflects a picture more complex than would be expected from a global assumption that stress causes sympathetic activation. For example, several physiological systems were measured among DSM-III-R GAD female clients and nonanxious controls during baseline rest and cognitive stress tests (Hoehn-Saric, McLeod, & Zimmerli, 1988b). Elevated muscle tension was found in the client group during rest, but no other measure distinguished the two groups. During stress, GAD clients showed stronger muscle tension response, but weaker skin conductance response and less variability in skin conductance and heart rate. These findings were in agreement with an earlier study using retrospective classification of subjects as having GAD (Hoehn-Saric & Masek, 1981), and led the authors to hypothesize that GAD clients are characterized by *inhibition* of some sympathetic systems and decreased autonomic flexibility. Normals, on the other hand, show stronger autonomic responses to stimuli, return to lower levels more quickly, and habituate faster (Lader & Wing, 1964) than do generally anxious clients, thus demonstrating greater autonomic flexibility.

Panic disorder clients have been found to show higher resting physiological activation than DSM-III GAD clients (Barlow et al., 1984), and greater resting heart rate and lower resting carbon dioxide pressure (pCO_2) than DSM-III GAD clients who had never experienced a panic attack (Rapee, 1986). However, the pCO_2 difference has not been replicated among DSM-III (Holt & Andrews, 1989) or DSM-III-R (de Ruiter et al., 1989) anxiety disorder groups, although agoraphobics with panic and panic disorder subjects did show elevated respiration relative to the combined group of social phobics and GAD clients in the latter study. Although no differences were found between DSM-III GAD and panic disorder clients on physiological meaures in another study (Borkovec & Mathews, 1988), greater cognitive (as opposed to somatic) symptomatology was related to (1) less heart rate reactivity to fearful imagery and physical exercise, (2) less respiration response to exercise, and (3) lower variability of heart rate during mental arithmetic.

Conclusions and Recommendations for Further Research

A few tentative conclusions are possible from the clinical studies described above. Unfortunately, such a limited data base exists that any conclusions can be seen only as potentially fruitful guides for future research into dimensions of pathological worry.

1. Interviewers can reliably agree on classification of 74–94% of reported worries into a small number of spheres. However, other findings in regard to content are less clear. First, the most frequent worry topics for GAD clients tend to vary somewhat from sample to sample, just as they do among normals, and no clear pattern emerges when spheres of normal versus GAD worry are compared. Second, the content of many worries does not fall neatly into the *a priori* categories employed thus far; there is a large miscellaneous category, perhaps larger among GAD than among control subjects, and possibly reflective of the greater variety of worrisome topics typical of these clients. Because GAD clients report more specific worries than nonanxious controls, the number of current worries may be a useful dimension of pathological worry to explore in the future. Third, no clinical study has examined change in worry content over time. If the focus of concern for GAD clients tends to be on variable, miscellaneous, and minor issues, the content should vary considerably from time to time and partly in response to life circumstances. Finally, there is reason to suspect the validity of the previously used categories. They are very global (e.g., family, interpersonal, finances), and particular worry content can be ambiguous with regard to the source of the worry, in cases where source would greatly influence classification. For example, a worry such as "I am concerned about the handling of family finances" may represent a true financial worry, a family/interpersonal worry if the client fears his or her spouse's evaluation of the financial handling, or both.

2. Most encouraging, though based on only one study, is the finding that independent interviewers can agree quite well on whether a client's worrying is excessive and/or unrealistic; thus, they appear to be responding to some as yet unspecified dimensions of worry report. GAD clients also characterize their worries as significantly more unrealistic than do nonanxious controls, and themselves as excessively worried about minor things. The latter results clearly distinguish the GAD group (91% and 93.6% in two studies) from other anxiety disorder groups (32% and 71%) and nonanxious controls (0%), although the test–retest report of clients is not perfect. Identification and quantification of whatever dimensions both interviewers and clients are using to make their judgments, as well as more standardized, elaborated ways of asking this question (to improve the clients' understanding

of the question and thus the reliability of their responses), may lead us to a more valid definition of pathological worry. Some limited evidence suggests what some of those dimensions may be, as discussed below.

GAD clients report feeling tense, anxious, and worried substantially more frequently than do nonanxious controls. In one study, a report of such feelings during 40% or more of the typical day identified all but 1 of 22 clients. Frequency was one of the distinguishing features of normal worries and intrusive thoughts, as reviewed earlier. Unfortunately, no data solely on the amount of worry, as opposed to tension and anxiety, have been collected on GAD samples, and no comparisons to other anxiety disorder groups have been made. Future research would usefully ask for frequency information on worry, tension, and anxiety separately; would obtain such frequency information from both GAD and other anxiety disorder groups; and would assess frequencies both when excluding and including worry about the central feature of other anxiety disorders.

4. The uncontrollability of worry may be its prime pathological feature. However, only a single clinical study (Craske et al., 1989) has addressed this issue: GAD clients report fewer obvious triggers to the initiation of their worrying, rate its controllability (once initiated) as lower, and report less success in applying methods to terminate the worrying than do control subjects. The centrality of the controllability dimension has been identified in the review of research on normal worries as well. Further work on measuring the uncontrollability of worry and contrasting GAD to other diagnostic groups would seem to be particularly promising.

5. Assessors do give GAD clients higher intensity ratings than some other anxiety disorder groups on the Hamilton items relating to cognitive anxiety symptoms. In one study looking at naturally occurring worry, GAD and nonanxious subjects did not differ; when asked about "significant" or "definite" worrying, all felt that the content produced equivalent anxiousness. This result parallels the finding in normal worry research that nonworriers will produce worry process similar in kind to that of worriers when the former are induced into a worrisome or anxious state, yet will show lower levels of intrusion than worriers at other times. Intensity, independent of frequency or uncontrollability, may not be a useful dimension for distinguishing between normal and pathological worry.

6. Because of the general absence of resources in clinical situations to measure the subtle preattentive bias toward threat found to be characteristic of GAD (see Chapter 4), it may be more useful in the future to develop methods of interview and self-report assessment that specifically address the ways in which and the degree to which worry interferes with a client's daily functioning. Promising preliminary results suggest that assessor ratings of interference may discriminate GAD from other anxiety disorders, although

separation of the effects of "anxiety" and "tension" from "worry" needs to be done, and larger samples of clients with the other disorders need to be acquired.

7. The partial separateness of worry from its somatic aspects has been shown in several studies of GAD clients for both perceived and actual physiological activity, paralleling findings with normal worry. However, except for the possibility that GAD involves inhibition of some sympathetic responses to stress, no somatic feature has emerged as uniquely characteristic of GAD relative to other anxiety disorders.

8. When research on normal and GAD worry (based on limited data) is compared, it does appear that worry in GAD involves an excess of the same process found in normals. However, insufficient data have been collected in clinical samples to allow determination of thresholds necessary for GAD diagnosis on the basis of promising dimensions of worry, such as uncontrollability, frequency, and interference. Systematic work on these dimensions may ultimately provide useful criteria for determining thresholds for pathological worry.

A THEORETICAL MODEL OF THE WORRY PROCESS

The chapter up to this point has reviewed much of the extant literature on worry-like phenomena; it indicates that a great deal remains to be learned about the worry process. However, recent experimental findings, combined with the largely descriptive research reviewed already, lead to some interesting possibilities for understanding the nature and function of worry. We argue that worry reflects the evolution of a conceptual avoidance response to perceived threat and contributes significantly to the maintenance of anxiety disorders. Some individuals, especially GAD clients, have come to depend on conceptual activity as the predominant mode of coping with their world, just as others depend primarily on overt motor avoidance, somatization, or some other protective defensive response.

Regardless of such individual differences, anxiety in any of its disorders is usefully viewed as a spiraling process of interaction over time among various internal human systems, including the conceptual, imaginal, affective–physiological, and behavioral channels. Each time a threat stimulus is perceived, defensive reactions are initiated, including autonomic activation and/or inhibition, behavioral avoidance and/or inhibition, catastrophic images, and catastrophic thinking. These reactions interact with each other, producing an increase in "anxiety" until the source of the threat is removed. Once the individual is out of danger, the entire episode with its sequential multichannel response events and behavioral and environmental consequences is stored in memory, further strengthening the associative network (Bower, 1981) that interconnects the various stimulus and response elements comprising the meaning of the event. The existence of such networks, strengthened by habitual modes of responding each time the threat is perceived, serves to prime the individual to detect such threat cues rapidly (even preattentively, outside of awareness), and to continue to generate interacting spirals of responses in a habitual, nonflexible way upon each detection of a threat (see Chapter 4).

Our theoretical model of worry suggests that within this generic model of anxiety, individual differences in certain of its elements yield the development and maintenance of GAD. The propositions of this model derive partly from the research reviewed earlier, but most importantly from recent studies described below.

Convincing evidence that worry is primariliy a conceptual process, and hints that this process may lead to an actual suppression of imagery, come from the following study (Borkovec & Inz, 1990). Thirteen DSM-III-R GAD clients, dual-diagnosed by separate interviewers on the ADIS-R, and 13 matched nonanxious controls underwent a 10-minute self-relaxation period and a 10-minute period of worrying about a topic of current concern. Mentation samples were obtained at three moments during each period. The degree of self-rated anxious valence of the mentations was greater for GAD clients than for controls throughout the relaxation and worry periods, although greater anxious valence occurred during worry than during self-relaxation. More importantly, clear differences in the occurrence of thinking versus imagery were found between groups and over periods. During relaxation, controls reported a predominance of imagery with little thought (56% vs. 15%), whereas GAD clients reported equivalent amounts of imagery and thought (36% vs. 33%). During worry, controls showed a predominance of thought over imagery (44% vs. 26%), with GAD clients reporting a further increase in thought (38%) and reduction of imagery (20%). Thus, worry is primarily a conceptual, verbal/linguistic activity. The amount of imagery declined among subjects in this order: relaxed nonanxious subjects, relaxed GADs, worrying nonanxious subjects, and worrying GADs. Although, descriptively, these results indicate a reduction in imagery over this dimension, there is reason to suspect that it may involve a *suppression* of imagery. Consider the following speculations and empirical support:

GAD clients have learned to emphasize conceptual activity as a primary mode of responding to perceived threat. Many chronic worriers report that they worry in order to anticipate and to avoid future catastrophes. Thus, worry may be a general example of long-term cognitive avoidance. However, their report may simply reflect an attempt to provide an explanation for an otherwise inexplicable and troublesome activity. The most exciting possibility emerging from recent research is that worry may be directly, immediately, and negatively reinforced by the avoidance of imagery, and therefore (Foa & Kozak, 1986; Lang, 1985) of peripheral physiological activation. GAD clients fear negative somatic arousal and affect. In response to perceived threat, the shifting of attention to conceptual activity at the very least reduces the available attentional resources that can be devoted to extant somatic–affective responses. But we are suggesting more than this. The active generation of worrisome conceptual activity reduces the generation of imagery and/or other routes to accessing memory structures that might otherwise issue efferent command into the autonomic and affective systems. We are positing an actual suppression of physiological–affective processes as a direct consequence of worrisome conceptual activity. One worries in order to avoid imagery and efferent command, and thus in order to avoid negative affect at the somatic level. There is a consequential increase in cortical activity and decrease in somatic activity. Such a model nicely subsumes a variety of data reviewed earlier:

1. GAD clients show signs of sympathetic inhibition and autonomic rigidity when stressed.
2. Greater cognitive (relative to somatic) symptomatology among GAD and panic clients is associated with less autonomic reactivity and variability in response to stress.
3. Worriers and nonworriers do not differ in peripheral physiological activation, either at rest or during worrying.
4. Worriers and nonworriers both show activation of the frontal cortex during worrying, with worriers showing greater left than right frontal activation compared to nonworriers.
5. GAD clients and chronic worriers report only modest somatic activation when anxious.

A final piece of evidence of this type was recently obtained by our research group: 200 undergraduates indicated how many DSM-III-R GAD somatic symptoms they commonly experienced whenever they felt anxious, as well as the percentage of thought versus the percentage of imagery they noticed when they worried. On the average, 70% of worry experience was reported to be composed of thought, whereas only 30% involved images. Most importantly, a significant negative correlation between amount of thought during worry and the number of indicated somatic symptoms was found. Thus, the more worry involves thought, the less somatic activation is reported. Worry thus leads to the suppression of imagery; imagery is the most potent internal route to, or reflection of, memory representational links to affective—physiological response; thus, worry provides for the avoidance of aversive somatic states.

Habitual behaviors are difficult to change, and hence are "uncontrollable," when they are supported by immediate reinforcement and there are punishing consequences for terminating the behavior. So, hypothetically, worry is uncontrollable, frequent, and intense because it is immediately reinforced (outside of the awareness of the individual) by suppression of somatic anxiety.

Equally exciting is the discovery that worry may maintain an anxiety disorder through its effects on a very fundamental process necessary for change in the dynamic human system. In the conceptual context of worrisome thinking, some information, especially emotional information, is not processed; thus, change is precluded. This conclusion is derived from a recent study that examined cardiovascular response to repeated phobic imagery (Borkovec & Hu, 1990). Subjects who thought about relaxing situations just before each image presentation displayed a customarily large heart rate reaction to the images, indicating that emotional processing was taking place. Subjects who thought about neutral situations showed significantly less reaction, whereas subjects who engaged in worrisome thinking displayed virtually no cardiovascular response to the images at all. Obviously, if one is attending excessively to negative thinking, fewer attentional resources can be devoted to the processing of new, immediately present, corrective information from the environment. But again, we are suggesting something even more active and fundamental, since all three groups in this study were engaging in thinking just before image onsets. The presence of excessive *worrisome* conceptual activity inhibits the complete accessing of fear structures from memory; without the recruitment of sufficient associative network links, including the apparently crucial response propositions and their efferent commands to the peripheral physiological—affective systems, emotional processing and its consequential modification of fear structure cannot take place (Foa & Kozak, 1986). Thus, worrying before, during, or after exposure to anxiety-relevant information can potentially retard or completely preclude extinction through repeated exposure. This is the third example of empirically documented cognitive avoidance effects. In the first example, attentional avoidance during exposure has been shown to inhibit therapeutic change in exposure treatment of anxiety disorders (Grayson, Foa, & Steketee, 1982, 1986; Sartory, Rachman, & Grey, 1982). In the second example, imagining an avoidance response to a feared situation after imaginal exposure to that situation has been demonstrated to maintain fear, despite otherwise sufficient amounts of exposure for producing change (Borkovec, 1974; Grayson & Borkovec, 1978). The third example (the Borkovec and Hu study) demonstrates that worrisome conceptual activity, by its hypothetical avoidance of imagery and affect, prevents the processing of information at these other, crucial levels of interacting multisystem process.

One can build a case for the mechanisms of this distinctive effect of worrisome conceptual activity, either from the behavioral inhibition theory of anxiety or from basic research in cognitive psychology. Gray (1982) argues that anxiety occurs either when expected information is aversive or when there is a mismatch between information expected and information received. In a relaxed state, the onset of a phobic image results in both conditions: It is aversive, and it creates a mismatch of information at the moment of image generation. The strong cardiovascular response to the image in this case reflects a fuller processing of the emotional material present in the image. In the context of worrisome conceptual activity, on the other hand, the image remains aversive, but there is less mismatch between conceptually expected and imaginally presented information. At some processing level, the brain is metaphorically saying to itself that the image contains no new information; thus, there is no need to process the emotional information. In terms of cognitive research, Smith (1984) has demonstrated that semantic satiation of a word leads to its isolation from the rest of its associative network. Thus, as the worrier repeatedly thinks about concerns, repetitiously using habitual, salient words, these words become increasingly insulated from their associative links—most importantly, from those links having to do with imagery, efferent command, peripheral physiology, and affect. From either theoretical view, worry precludes the processing of information and thus maintains the anxiety disorder.

If it turns out that worry indeed does have such an effect on emotional processing, the implications would be potentially very important. At the theoretical level, we would begin to get hints about how the conceptual, verbal/linguistic system interacts with the other systems. Such basic knowledge could ultimately contribute to improvements in how cognitive therapy is conducted and how we might integrate cognitive methods with imaginal, behavioral, and affective techniques. At the pragmatic level, this hypothesized effect would suggest that individual differences in responsiveness to exposure techniques in all of the anxiety disorders, as well as the occurrence of maintenance or relapse, may reflect the degree to which certain types of conceptual activity are working against the therapeutic change process that is otherwise inherent in exposure methods. In addition, for GAD, there would be the pragmatic suggestion that repeated exposure to imagery and affect may be a particularly important technique for overcoming the inherently avoidant process of worry.

Etiological questions are always difficult to address in a convincing fashion, but some of the extant research on worry suggests possible hints about how one might develop chronic worry. Degree of worry correlates most highly with social-evaluative fears (e.g., fear of criticism, fear of making mistakes, and fear of meeting someone for the first time). Moreover, social phobia is a very common secondary diagnosis for GADs (59%; Barlow, 1988). It is also useful to realize that the verbal/linguistic system evolved fundamentally as a social device; that is, symbols representing concrete objects or actions were used to communicate information to other humans. The origins of thinking ("talking to ourselves") reside developmentally and evolutionarily in talking to others. Thus thinking is an inherently social process and may be speculatively viewed as talking to representations of others from our past and current lives. When we are engaged in problem solving, for example, the developmental prototype involves reasoning with parents or teachers. When we are worrying about the future, the prototype involves expressing our fears to those in our childhood world to whom we turned for reassurance, support, or solution. When we ruminate about a past transgression, the prototype is our verbal expression of feared loss, guilt, rationalization, or defensive argument to those against whom we transgressed. The combination of social fear in worry, fear and avoidance of somatic anxiety, and the social origins of thought suggests that chronic worriers may have a history of aversive events associated with other people, especially events having to do with emotional expression, the potential loss of love or approval, and the use of internal and external language to try to cope with these.

Finally, the various pieces of empirical information provide some understanding for the variability of spheres of worry and diffuse nature of GAD. Frequent rehearsal of negative associations at the conceptual level (worry) primes preattentive bias to threat cues (see Chapter 4). The strong contribution of social-evaluative fears to worry guarantees that many life circumstances can pose threats to the adequacy of one's anticipated performances, circumstances, and self-concept. If what one often fears is the making of mistakes, virtually any demanding environmental event—especially social events where public detection of mistakes is possible—is a potential danger. What worries a person in the moment depends on what life events are present or approaching. Not only will many environmental cues thus be primed by worrisome conceptual activity, but there may be strong links among different worry spheres. R. L. Metzger (personal communication, 1990) has recently demonstrated that worry serves as a superordinate category: The activation of one worry sphere spreads to other, content-unrelated worry spheres, such that information relevant to those other spheres is more rapidly processed even though the spheres themselves were not directly primed. Thus worrisome activity is likely to involve movement of thinking across different spheres of current concern, and is also triggered by many potential cues.

Conceptual processes reflect perhaps the crowning achievement of human evolution. They provide greater freedom of response from the environment, with opportunities to explore and experiment with what might be or can be. With this advantage comes potential disadvantages: an overdependence on abstract processes that may bear little connection to what actually is or probably will be, and, in the case of worry, a predominance of negatively valenced thought. The consequence appears to be a reduction in new learning and the maintenance of distressing emotional states. It is important, therefore, that we continue to pursue how human conceptual activity influences and is affected by other levels of system functioning in general, and how worrisome thought in particular can best be modified to remove its maintaining effects on emotional disorders.

Acknowledgment. Preparation of this chapter was supported in part by Research Grant No. MH-39172 to Thomas D. Borkovec from the National Institute of Mental Health.

REFERENCES

Barlow, D. H. (1988). *Anxiety and its disorders: The nature and treatment of anxiety and panic.* New York: Guilford Press.

Barlow, D. H., Blanchard, E. B., Vermilyea, J. A., Vermilyea, B. B., & Di Nardo, P. A. (1986). Generalized anxiety and generalized anxiety disorder: Description and reconceptualization. *American Journal of Psychiatry, 143,* 40–44.

Barlow, D. H., Cohen, A. D., Waddell, M. T., Vermilyea, B. B., Klosko, J. S., Blanchard, E. B., & Di Nardo, P. A. (1984). Panic and generalized anxiety disorders: Nature and treatment. *Behavior Therapy, 15,* 431–449.

Borkovec, T. D. (1974). Heart rate process during systematic desensitization and implosive therapy for analogue anxiety. *Behavior Therapy, 5,* 636–641.

Borkovec, T. D., & Hu, S. (1990). The effect of worry on cardiovascular response to phobic imagery. *Behaviour Research and Therapy, 28,* 69–73.

Borkovec, T. D., & Inz, J. (1990). The nature of worry in generalized anxiety disorder: A predominance of thought activity. *Behaviour Research and Therapy, 28,* 153–158.

Borkovec, T. D., & Mathews, A. M. (1988). Treatment of non-phobic anxiety disorders: A comparison of nondirective, cognitive, and coping desensitization therapy. *Journal of Consulting and Clinical Psychology, 56,* 877–884.

Borkovec, T. D., Robinson, E., Pruzinsky, T., & DePree, J. A. (1983). Preliminary exploration of worry: Some characteristics and processes. *Behaviour Research and Therapy, 21,* 9–16.

Bower, G. H. (1981). Mood and memory. *American Psychologist, 36,* 129–148.

Carter, W. R., Johnson, M. C., & Borkovec, T. D. (1986). Worry: An electrocortical analysis. *Advances in Behaviour Research and Therapy, 8,* 193–204.

Clark, D. A. (1986). Factors influencing the retrieval and control of negative cognitions. *Behaviour Research and Therapy*, *24*, 151–159.

Clark, D. A., & de Silva, P. (1985). The nature of depressive and anxious, intrusive thoughts: Distinct or uniform phenomena? *Behaviour Research and Therapy*, *23*, 383–393.

Craske, M. G., Rapee, R. M., Jackel, L., & Barlow, D. H. (1989). Qualitative dimensions of worry in DSM-III-R generalized anxiety disorder subjects and nonanxious controls. *Behaviour Research and Therapy*, *27*, 397–402.

Deffenbacher, J. L. (1977). Relationship of worry and emotionality to performance on the Miller Analogies Test. *Journal of Educational Psychology*, *69*, 191–195.

Deffenbacher, J. L. (1980). Worry and emotionality in test anxiety. In I. G. Sarason (Ed.), *Test anxiety: Theory, research and application*. Hillside, NJ: Erlbaum.

Deffenbacher, J. L. (1986). Cognitive and physiological components of test anxiety in real-life exams. *Cognitive Therapy and Research*, *10*, 635–644.

de Ruiter, C., Garssen, B., Rijken, H., & Kraaimaat, F. (1989). The hyperventilation syndrome in panic disorder, agoraphobia and generalized anxiety disorder. *Behaviour Research and Therapy*, *27*, 447–452.

Di Nardo, P. A., & Barlow, D. H. (1988). *Anxiety Disorders Interview Schedule— Revised (ADIS-R)*. Albany: Center for Stress and Anxiety Disorders, University at Albany, State University of New York.

Di Nardo, P. A., & Barlow, D. H. (1990). Syndrome and symptom comorbidity in the anxiety disorders. In J. D. Maser & C. R. Cloninger (Eds.), *Comorbidity in anxiety and mood disorders*. Washington, DC: American Psychiatric Press.

Edwards, S., & Dickerson, M. (1987a). Intrusive unwanted thoughts: A two-stage model of control. *British Journal of Medical Psychology*, *60*, 317–328.

Edwards, S., & Dickerson, M. (1987b). On the similarity of positive and negative intrusions. *Behaviour Research and Therapy*, *25*, 207–211.

England, S. L., & Dickerson, M. (1988). Intrusive thoughts: Unpleasantness not the major cause of uncontrollability. *Behaviour Research and Therapy*, *26*, 279–282.

Eysenck, M. W. (1984). Anxiety and the worry process. *Bulletin of the Psychonomic Society*, *22*, 545–548.

Foa, E. B., & Kozak, M. J. (1986). Emotional processing of fear: Exposure to corrective information. *Psychological Bulletin*, *99*, 20–35.

Gray, J. A. (1982). Precis of "The neuropsychology of anxiety: An inquiry into the functions of the septo-hippocampal system." *Behavioral and Brain Sciences*, *5*, 469–534.

Grayson, J. B., & Borkovec, T. C. (1978). The effects of expectancy and imaged response to phobic stimuli on fear reduction. *Cognitive Therapy and Research*, *2*, 11–24.

Grayson, J. B., Foa, E. B., & Steketee, G. S. (1982). Habituation during exposure treatment: Distraction vs. attention-focusing. *Behaviour Research and Therapy*, *20*, 323–328.

Grayson, J. B., Foa, E. B., & Steketee, G. S. (1986). Exposure *in vivo* of obsessive–compulsives under distracting and attention-focusing conditions: Replication and extension. *Behaviour Research and Therapy*, *24*, 475–479.

Gross, P. R., Oei, T. P. S., & Evans, L. (1989). Generalized anxiety symptoms in phobic disorders and anxiety states: A test of the worry hypothesis. *Journal of Anxiety Disorders, 3,* 159–169.

Hatfield, B. D., Doyle, L. A., & Borkovec, T. D. (1981). *A validation of the Autonomic Perception Questionnaire with implications for sports anxiety management.* Monterey, CA: National Association for the Study of the Psychology of Sport and Physical Activity.

Hoehn-Saric, R., & Masek, B. J. (1981). Effects of naloxone on normals and chronically anxious patients. *Biological Psychiatry, 16,* 1041–1050.

Hoehn-Saric, R., & McLeod, D. R. (1988). The peripheral sympathetic nervous system: Its role in normal and pathologic anxiety. *Psychiatric Clinics of North America, 11,* 375–386.

Hoehn-Saric, R., McLeod, D., & Zimmerli, W. D. (1988a). Differential effects of alprazolam and imipramine in generalized anxiety disorder: Somatic versus psychic symptoms. *Journal of Clinical Psychiatry, 49,* 293–301.

Hoehn-Saric, R., McLeod, D. R., & Zimmerli, W. D. (1988b). *Subjective and somatic manifestations of anxiety in obsessive–compulsive and generalized anxiety disorders.* Paper presented at the 141st Annual Meeting of the American Psychiatric Association, Montreal.

Holt, P. E., & Andrews, G. (1989). Hyperventilation and anxiety in panic disorder, social phobia, GAD and normal controls. *Behaviour Research and Therapy, 27,* 453–460.

Karteroliotis, C., & Gill, D. L. (1987). Temporal changes in psychological and physiological components of state anxiety. *Journal of Sport Psychology, 9,* 261–274.

Kent, G., & Jambunathan, P. (1989). A longitudinal study of the intrusiveness of cognitions in test anxiety. *Behaviour Research and Therapy, 27,* 43–50.

Lader, M. H., & Wing, L. (1964). Habituation of the psychogalvanic reflex in patients with anxiety states and in normal subjects. *Journal of Neurology, Neurosurgery and Psychiatry, 27,* 210–218.

Lang, P. J. (1985). The cognitive psychophysiology of emotion: Fear and anxiety. In A. H. Tuma & J. Maser (Eds.), *Anxiety and the anxiety disorders.* Hillsdale, NJ: Erlbaum.

Levy, S., & Guttman, L. (1976). Worry, fear, and concern differentiated. *Israel Annals of Psychiatry and Related Disciplines, 14,* 211–228.

McCarthy, P. R., & Borkovec, T. C. (1983). *Worry: Basic characteristics and processes.* Paper presented at the meeting of the Association for Advancement of Behavior Therapy, Washington, DC.

McLeod, D. R., Hoehn-Saric, R., & Stefan, R. L. (1986). Somatic symptoms of anxiety: Comparison of self-report and physiological measures. *Biological Psychiatry, 21,* 301–310.

Metzger, R. L., Miller, M., Cohen, M., Sofka, M., & Borkovec, T. D. (1990). Worry changes decision making: The effect of negative thoughts on cognitive processing. *Journal of Clinical Psychology, 46,* 78–88.

Morris, L. W., Davis, M. A., & Hutchings, C. H. (1981). Cognitive and emotional components of anxiety: Literature review and a revised worry–emotionality scale. *Journal of Educational Psychology*, *73*, 541–555.

Parkinson, L., & Rachman, S. (1981). Part II: The nature of intrusive thoughts. *Advances in Behaviour Research and Therapy*, *3*, 101–110.

Rapee, R. (1986). Differential response to hyperventilation in panic disorder and generalized anxiety disorder. *Journal of Abnormal Psychology*, *95*, 24–28.

Salkovskis, P. M., & Harrison, J. (1984). Abnormal and normal obsessions: A replication. *Behaviour Research and Therapy*, *22*, 549–552.

Sanderson, W. C., & Barlow, D. H. (1990). A description of patients diagnosed with DSM-III revised generalized anxiety disorder. *Journal of Nervous and Mental Diseases*, *178*, 588–591.

Sarason, I. G., Sarason, B. R., Keefe, D. E., Hayes, B. E., & Shearin, E. N. (1986). Cognitive interference: Situational determinants and traitlike characteristics. *Journal of Personality and Social Psychology*, *51*, 215–226.

Sartory, G., Rachman, S., & Grey, S. J. (1982). Return of fear: The role of rehearsal. *Behaviour Research and Therapy*, *20*, 123–133.

Simon, A., & Ward, L. O. (1974). Variables influencing the sources, frequency and intensity of worry in secondary school pupils. *British Journal of Social and Clinical Psychology*, *13*, 391–396.

Simon, A., & Ward, L. O. (1982). Sex-related patterns of worry in secondary school pupils. *British Journal of Clinical Psychology*, *21*, 63–64.

Smith, L. C. (1984). Semantic satiation affects category membership decision time but not lexical priming. *Memory and Cognition*, *12*, 483–488.

Sutherland, G., Newman, B., & Rachman, S. (1982). Experimental investigations of the relations between mood and intrusive unwanted cognitions. *British Journal of Medical Psychology*, *55*, 127–138.

Wisocki, P. A. (1988). Worry as a phenomenon relevant to the elderly. *Behavior Therapy*, *19*, 369–379.

York, D., Borkovec, T. D., Vasey, M., & Stern, R. (1987). Effects of worry and somatic anxiety induction on thoughts, emotion and physiological activity. *Behaviour Research and Therapy*, *25*, 523–526.

3

The Biology of Generalized Anxiety Disorder and Chronic Anxiety

DEBORAH S. COWLEY
PETER P. ROY-BYRNE
University of Washington School of Medicine

I n 1980, with the publication of the *Diagnostic and Statistical Manual of Mental Disorders*, third edition (DSM-III), anxiety neurosis was divided into generalized anxiety disorder (GAD) and panic disorder. Since then, the biology of panic disorder has been the subject of considerable research interest (reviewed in Roy-Byrne & Cowley, 1988). By contrast, GAD has been relatively neglected.

This neglect has stemmed in part from the heterogeneity of patients with GAD. The definition of GAD has changed significantly during the last 10 years; interrater reliability for diagnosis of GAD is lower than for other anxiety disorders (Di Nardo, O'Brien, Barlow, Waddell, & Blanchard, 1983); and the boundary between GAD and normal anxiety or adjustment reactions is unclear. GAD coexists with many other psychiatric disorders (Barlow, Blanchard, Vermilyea, Vermilyea, & Di Nardo, 1986; Breier, Charney, & Heninger, 1985) and may, when made as a cross-sectional diagnosis, actually represent a residual or prodromal form of another disorder, especially major depression or panic disorder. Patients with subthreshold forms of obsessive compulsive disorder, social phobia, panic disorder, or adult forms of attention deficit disorder may be given a diagnosis of GAD. Unidentified alcohol or substance abuse or dependence is often mistaken for GAD, especially when no obvious evidence of significant familial, occupational, or social dysfunction is present. On the other hand, some writers have pointed out that chronic pathological anxiety, or GAD, may be the core underlying disorder in many patients and may predispose them to superimposed, more circumscribed episodes of affective or anxiety disorders (e.g., Tyrer, 1985).

This diagnostic confusion makes the identification of relatively homogeneous groups for biological studies difficult. Furthermore, the vague amorphous nature of "generalized anxiety" has been less attractive to biological researchers than the discrete, dramatic phenomenon of a panic attack. Despite this, several studies over the past few years have examined biological aspects of GAD. In this chapter, we review current knowledge of the biology of GAD. Although we emphasize those recent studies using DSM-III or DSM-III-R diagnostic criteria, we also summarize major findings from earlier investigations of the biology of chronic anxiety.

THE BIOLOGY OF "STRESS" IN NORMAL VOLUNTEERS

Chronic "pathological" anxiety has long been considered an extension of the normal stress response. An extensive literature attests to the significant physiological and hormonal changes accompanying acute psychological stress in normal volunteers (for reviews, see Lader, 1980; Rose, 1984). Chronically anxious patients complain of many symptoms characteristic of acute stress-induced anxiety, such as palpitations, muscle tension, tremor, sweating, and gastrointestinal distress. For this reason, investigations of the biology of chronic anxiety states have generally been based on those of normal stress, and have used similar paradigms and measures. We briefly review the methods and general results of these studies in normals as a background to our discussion of findings in chronically anxious patients.

The effects of psychological stress on healthy volunteers have been studied both in natural situations (e.g., academic examinations, anticipation of surgery, work settings, military combat, or parachute training) and in the laboratory. Laboratory paradigms have included stressful interviews, loud noises, mental arithmetic, cold pressor tests, films of distasteful scenes, and anticipation of painful stimuli such as electric shocks. These studies have all examined the effects of an externally applied "stressor" assumed to be universally anxiety-provoking to healthy subjects. However, although most of these stressors are accompanied by increased arousal, the amount and type of anxiety experienced by the individual subject—and thus presumably the magnitude and type of biological changes observed—clearly depend on the meaning of the situation and the degree of threat that it poses for that subject (Rose, 1984; Hoehn-Saric & McLeod, 1988).

Responses to stress may also differ with genetic predisposition, affective state, and personality. For example, normotensive subjects with a family history of hypertension show greater blood pressure and cortisol, but not skin conductance, responses to mental stress than subjects without such a family history (Hoehn-Saric & McLeod, 1988). Heightened affect, especially anxiety or hostility, has been associated with greater 17-hydroxycorticosteroid excretion with stress (Curtis, Fogel, McEvoy, & Zarate, 1970), whereas subjects with depressive tendencies displayed a reduced epinephrine response during mental tasks when compared with other subjects (Frankenhaeuser & Patkai, 1965).

Given the multiple factors influencing the affective and biological responses of a given person to a specific testing situation, it is not surprising that studies of the effects of acute stress often yield inconsistent results (see Lader, 1980; Rose, 1984). Neuroendocrine measures appear particularly variable. Cortisol levels are affected by diurnal variation, whereas growth hormone responses to stress may depend on stimulus intensity and the pulsatile, intermittent nature of growth hormone secretion. Catecholamines show marked responsivity to a wide variety of stimuli, such as postural changes, venipuncture, obesity, and eating. Assays for catecholamine levels have until recently shown significant variability. These methodological factors make it difficult to interpret many catecholamine studies, especially those attempting to link epinephrine release with novel situations and norepinephrine release with vigilance or effort (Rose, 1984).

Despite all of these sources of individual response variability, however, most of these studies suggest that healthy subjects under stress display evidence of increased arousal, including increased heart rate, blood pressure, respiration, and muscle tension. Both skin conductance levels and the number of spontaneous fluctuations increase (Hoehn-Saric & McLeod, 1988). Vascular changes include cutaneous vasoconstriction and vasodilation in striate muscles. Hormonally, levels of circulating catecholamines, cortisol, prolactin, growth hormone, and free fatty acids increase (Lader, 1980; Rose, 1984).

It is important to note that these changes are not unique to anxiety-provoking situations, but are also observed in subjects reporting anger, fear, or intense pleasure. They are thus likely to reflect nonspecific states of arousal. It remains unclear how arousal-related biological changes are related to the cognitive experience of anxiety in normals or in patients with anxiety disorders, and whether other, more specific biological abnormalities might give rise to particular forms of pathological anxiety.

There is relatively little information regarding the effects of chronic stress, a situation potentially of more relevance to chronic anxiety disorders. However, several studies suggest that both animals and humans display habituation after repeated exposure to a novel, stressful stimulus or task (Rose, 1984; Lader & Wing, 1964). Habituation may be more rapid for adrenocortical responses than for catecholamine release, and responses to other acute stressors may be unchanged or more pronounced.

THE BIOLOGY OF CHRONIC ANXIETY

Before 1980, studies of the biology of chronic anxiety disorders suffered not only from the sources of variability noted above, but also from the use of a wide variety of patient groups—from "psychoneurotics" with neurasthenia, anxiety neurosis, or psychasthenia, to general psychiatric patients with an assortment of primary diagnoses but prominent anxiety symptoms. No doubt as a result of these mixed patient groups, these studies often yielded disparate results. For example, when compared with normal controls, patients displayed elevated or normal resting heart rates and increased, decreased, or similar levels of skin conductance. Despite this, these studies do suggest that patients with chronic anxiety show characteristic response patterns that are not merely an exaggeration of the normal stress response.

Neuroendocrine Findings

Psychiatric patients with high anxiety ratings or in acute anxiety states were found in several studies to have elevated resting plasma cortisol, plasma adrenocorticotropin (ACTH), and urinary 17-hydroxycorticosteroids (Bliss, Migeon, Branch, & Samuels, 1956; Persky et al., 1956). Patients were also more likely than controls to show fluctuations in urinary 17-hydroxycorticosteroids according to the intensity of their mood, and higher urinary corticosteroid levels following ACTH administration (Persky, 1957). Neurotic patients had greater cortisol and growth hormone responses than controls to a mirror drawing test (Miyabo, Hisada, Asato, Mizushima, & Ueno, 1976).

One study (Reiss et al., 1951) found decreased thyroid function, as measured by radioactive iodine uptake, in anxious men, but increased thyroid function in anxious women. However, Dongier, Wittkower, Stephens-Newsham, and Hoffman (1956) found no relationship between anxiety level and thyroid function in a group of 71 anxious patients. Prolactin levels, although sometimes elevated with stress, showed no change in one study of relaxation treatment of generalized anxiety (Mathew, Ho, Kralik, & Claghorn, 1979).

Catecholamines

Surprisingly few studies of catecholamine function in anxiety disorders were performed prior to 1980. In one study of inpatients with both anxiety and depression, catecholamine levels were elevated and correlated with anxiety but not depression scores (Wyatt, Porkorny, Kupfer, Snyder, & Engelman, 1971). The catecholamine metabolites metadrenaline and nor-metadrenaline were found to be elevated in psychiatric inpatients during periods of agitation (Nelson, Masuda, & Holmes, 1966). Administration of catecholamines (particularly epinephrine) induced typical physical, but not emotional, symptoms ("cold fear") in subjects with anxiety disorders. Free fatty acid levels, an indirect measure of catecholamine release, were correlated with the anxiety content of speech in psychiatric patients (Gotts-chalk, Cleghorn, Gleser, & Iacono, 1965). In several studies using stress procedures, however, "neurotic" subjects displayed weaker catecholamine responses than subjects with "stable personalities," and showed delayed recovery of catecholamine levels to baseline (Frankenhaeuser, 1979; Frosman, 1980).

Psychophysiology

As noted above, resting heart rate was observed to be elevated or normal in anxious patients. Blood pressure was found to be elevated and more labile (Lader, 1980). On a cold pressor test, a group of patients with anxiety neurosis showed prolonged increases in blood pressure, with delayed adaptation to the stress procedure as compared with controls (Malmo, Shagass, & Heslam, 1951). Similarly, patients displayed significant delays in recovery of pupil size to baseline after a cold pressor test, although no patient–control differences in pupil size were noted at baseline or during the stress (Rubin, 1964).

As also mentioned above, the resting levels of skin conductance in anxious patients were found to vary considerably, with different studies showing elevations, no patient–control differences, or decreases. However, the bulk of studies showed increased resting levels with higher spontaneous fluctuation rates (Lader, 1980; Hoehn-Saric & McLeod, 1988). On stressful tasks, patients appeared to show changes in both absolute levels and fluc-tuation rates that were identical to or less pronounced than those of controls. Impaired habituation of skin conductance responses was noted in several studies of anxious patients, with anxiety levels being correlated with the degree of delay in habituation (Lader & Wing, 1964; Lader, 1967). Delayed habituation and high spontaneous fluctuation rates in skin conductance were associated with a poor response to systematic desensitization (Lader, Gelder, & Marks, 1967).

Forearm blood flow was increased at rest in one study of anxiety neurotics (Kelly, Brown, & Shaffer, 1970); however, patients showed a less pronounced response on a mental arithmetic task, with both groups increasing to the same value. Psychoneurotics were found to show significant cutaneous vasoconstriction while awake, with marked vasodilation during sleep (Ackner, 1956).

Electromyographic (EMG) studies generally showed increased EMG activity, and thus muscle tension, in anxious patients when compared to controls, both at rest and during stressful stimuli (Lader, 1980). However, there was considerable variation between studies in the particular muscle groups showing patient–control differences, with the frontalis muscle the most consistently different. Some of the variability in results may have been due to differences between those anxious patients with and those without muscle tension symptoms in particular muscle groups. Tense patients also showed less habituation of EMG responses on retrial than controls.

Anxious patients consistently showed electroencephalographic (EEG) changes, including increased beta and decreased alpha activity; increased harmonic driving of the EEG by photic stimulation was also correlated with anxiety levels (Lader, 1980). The contingent negative variation (CNV) or expectancy wave, an EEG response to anticipation of a stimulus, was decreased in anxious patients versus controls, implying greater distractibility. Patients also showed impaired habituation of CNV.

Anxious patients have also been noted to have increased respiratory rates. In fact, anxiety disorders have been linked with the hyperventilation syndrome. Both acute hyperventilation and the chronic hyperventilation syndrome are associated with, and have recently been examined in patients with, panic disorder (for a review, see Cowley & Roy-Byrne, 1987). Several studies have also observed that stress or anxiety states could give rise to hyperventilation and that hyperventilation, once initiated, in turn worsened anxiety (Kerr, Dalton, & Gliebe, 1937; Lewis, 1954; Suess, Alexander, Sweeney, & Marion, 1980). Interestingly, patients with the chronic hyperventilation syndrome displayed delayed recovery of partial pressure of carbon dioxide (pCO_2) after acute overbreathing (Hardonk & Beumer, 1979).

With exercise, patients with neurocirculatory asthenia were found to have decreased exercise tolerance and increased lactate production (Jones & Mellersh, 1946; Cohen, Consolazio, & Johnson, 1947; Holmgren & Strom, 1959). This finding led to Pitts and McClure's (1967) discovery that intravenous sodium lactate infusion provoked panic and anxiety symptoms in patients with anxiety neurosis, and to the wide use of lactate infusion in research studies as a provocative test for panic.

Overall, studies of the biology of chronic anxiety conducted prior to 1980 suggested a state of heightened autonomic arousal at rest in anxious patients, with findings reminiscent of acute stress-induced anxiety in normals. However, anxious patients also displayed considerable inter- and intraindividual variability in most measures in the resting state. Their responses to stressful tasks or situations were often less marked than those of control subjects, although this may have represented a ceiling effect. One of the most consistent findings across variables was that of impaired habituation to repetitions of the same stimulus, with delayed recovery to a baseline state.

As discussed above, nonpsychiatric subjects generally show rapid habituation to repetitions of the same stimulus. The fact that chronically anxious patients continue to display resting autonomic arousal after years of illness suggests that these disorders are indeed quite different from the normal response to chronic stress and that the observed deficit in habituation may be a central part of the underlying pathophysiology of chronic anxiety disorders.

STUDIES OF PATIENTS WITH GAD

Since 1980, several biological studies have examined patients diagnosed as having GAD according to DSM-III or DSM-III-R criteria. Although the use of these standardized diagnostic criteria yields more homogeneous samples, it is important to keep in mind that the criteria changed with DSM-III-R, primarily in requiring a 6-month as opposed to a 1-month duration of illness. In addition, many of the biological studies to be discussed included patients with infrequent panic attacks and past major depression.

Studies of GAD have examined many of the endocrine and psychophysiological measures discussed above. In addition, some have looked at sleep, cerebral blood flow and metabolism, and specific neurotransmitter systems that may be involved in the pathophysiology of pathological anxiety. We discuss existing reports of neurotransmitter function in patients, as well as selected animal studies indicating promising areas of future investigation. Since genetic transmission of a disorder indicates that specific gene-encoded changes in proteins and the resulting biological abnormalities may be causal as opposed to resulting from or occurring with the illness, we also discuss the few available data from family studies of GAD.

Family Studies

Family and twin studies suggest a familial and probably a genetic basis for panic disorder (e.g., Crowe, Noyes, Pauls, & Slymen, 1983; Torgerson, 1983). Earlier findings of a familial aggregation of anxiety neurosis (Cohen, Badal, Kilpatrick, Reed, & White, 1951; Wheeler, White, Reed, & Cohen, 1948) may thus have been attributable to the familial transmission of panic attacks. However, an extensive animal and human literature (reviewed in Barlow, 1988) suggests that emotionality, "nervousness," neuroticism, and nonclinical anxiety are heritable. It seems likely that pathological generalized anxiety may also have a genetic component.

To date, only one study has specifically examined familial transmission of GAD (Noyes, Clarkson, Crowe, Yates, & McChesney, 1987). The 20 probands with DSM-III GAD had no history of panic attacks. Of 123 first-degree relatives of these probands, 24 (19.5%) met criteria for GAD, as opposed to 3.5% (4 of 113) of relatives of controls and 5.4% (13 of 241) of relatives of probands with panic disorder. Relatives of GAD probands had a mild and often stress-related form of GAD. Panic disorder was no more common in relatives of GAD patients than in relatives of controls, and was significantly less frequent than in relatives of panic disorder patients (4.1% vs. 14.9%). The major limitation of this study is that diagnoses of relatives were not made blindly. However, the results indicate that GAD can be distinguished from panic disorder on the basis of family history. Further studies are necessary to establish familial transmission of GAD.

Catecholamines

The few studies of catecholamines in GAD have unfortunately yielded inconclusive results. Resting levels of catecholamines and of their metabolite 3-methoxy-4-hydroxyphenethylene glycol (MHPG) have been noted by two groups (Mathew, Ho, et al., 1980; Sevy, Papadimitriou, Surmont, Goldman, & Mendlewicz, 1989) to be elevated in patients with GAD. However, a later study by Mathew, Ho, Francis, Taylor, and Weinman (1982) failed to replicate their earlier findings, which they suggested may have resulted from the stress of venipuncture. Another study (Munjack et al., 1990), in which blood was drawn after 20 minutes' rest through an indwelling catheter to control for the effects of venipuncture, showed no significant patient–control differences in resting epinephrine or norepinephrine. There was a small but significant increase in plasma MHPG in GAD patients, but on discriminant analysis this did not significantly predict diagnosis.

The differing results of these studies probably reflect methodological difficulties in studying catecholamines, as well as possible differences in patient populations or experimental settings. As noted, only the study of Munjack et al. (1990) controlled specifically for the effects of venipuncture. None of the studies controlled for diet or exercise level; moreover, all sampled venous blood, which introduces significant variability (especially in norepinephrine) as a result of extraction across the forearm venous bed (Best & Halter, 1982). In addition, catecholamine assays, although improved in reliability with recent radioenzymatic techniques, remain subject to considerable variability, and peripheral measurements of catecholamines and MHPG reflect both peripheral and central nervous system activity.

Sevy et al. (1989) also measured platelet alpha-2-adrenoreceptor binding, using yohimbine (an alpha-2 antagonist) as a ligand; they found a lower calculated maximal number of binding sites, and thus presumably a decrease in receptor number, in GAD patients than in controls and patients with major depression. Abelson et al. (1991) found a blunted growth hormone response to clonidine in GAD, a finding possibly consistent with that of Sevy et al. (1989) and suggesting perhaps subsensitivity of postsynaptic alpha-2 receptors. However, they did not note any patient–control differences in clonidine's effects on MHPG, blood pressure, heart rate, or self-rated sedation, and noted that their growth hormone finding could also be attributable to a blunted growth hormone response to growth-hormone-releasing hormone.

In contrast to these studies, Charney, Woods, and Heninger (1989) found no GAD–control differences in self-rated anxiety, cortisol, blood pressure, heart rate, or plasma MHPG after 20 mg of oral yohimbine. In fact, there was a trend for a less marked increase in MHPG in patients with GAD. Charney et al.'s findings clearly differentiate patients with GAD from those with panic disorder, about 50% of whom show increased self-rated anxiety, cortisol, MHPG, and cardiovascular responses to yohimbine (Charney, Heninger, & Breier, 1984).

Levels of catechol-O-methyl transferase and dopamine-beta-hydroxylase, two enzymes responsible for the degradation of catecholamines, showed no patient–control differences (Mathew, Ho, et al., 1980; Mathew, Ho, Taylor, & Semchuk, 1981). In one study, platelet monoamine oxidase (MAO) activity was elevated in anxious patients and then decreased during relaxation training (Mathew, Ho, Kralik, Weinman, & Claghorn, 1981). Another report showed no differences from controls in platelet MAO activity (Khan et al., 1986). As Khan et al. (1986) point out, the significant sex differences in platelet MAO levels and small numbers of subjects included in many studies may have confounded the results.

In sum, several reports suggest possible abnormalities in catecholamine function in GAD. However, such abnormalities do not appear to be a clear-cut or striking concomitant of pathological anxiety. This is surprising, given the association between stress and increased catecholamines, but may be due to the limitations of peripheral measurements in assessing central adrenergic function, to more subtle abnormalities in the adrenergic system and its responsiveness to stress in GAD, or to a different biological basis for GAD than for normal stress-induced arousal.

Neuroendocrine Findings

In contrast to earlier findings of increased cortisol in psychoneurotic patients, Rosenbaum et al. (1983) found no differences in basal urinary free cortisol in patients with GAD. Patients with GAD do, however, demonstrate an elevated dexamethasone suppression test nonsuppression rate (Avery et al., 1985; Schweizer, Swenson, Winokur, Rickels, & Maislin, 1986) of about 27–38% when a 4 mg/ml cutoff is used. This rate is clearly higher than that reported for panic disorder and similar to that found in outpatient major depression. Furthermore, nonsuppression in anxious patients was unrelated to Hamilton Rating Scale for Depression scores or to the presence of secondary depression (Avery et al., 1985). Tiller, Biddle, Maguire, and Davies (1988) found lower plasma dexamethasone levels in both GAD and control nonsuppressors. After treatment, patients with GAD were all suppressors, but those who had been nonsuppressors continued to display low plasma dexamathasone levels. The authors speculated that a low dexamethasone level may allow higher cortisol levels in the presence of higher state anxiety. Thus, there are indications of possible hypothalamic–pituitary–adrenal axis dysfunction in GAD and chronic anxiety; however, these are not uniformly supported and require further investigation.

Despite the possible association between hyperthyroidism and GAD (Kathol, Turner, & Delahunt, 1986), the one study of patients with GAD showed normal thyroid function, as measured by total serum thyroxine, free thyroxine index, triiodothyronine resin uptake, and thyroid-stimulating hormone (Munjack & Palmer, 1988).

Psychophysiology

The few psychophysiological studies of GAD have displayed no patient–control differences in electrodermal activity, respiration, blood pressure, or heart interbeat interval at rest (Hoehn-Saric & Masek, 1981); Hoehn-Saric, McLeod, & Zimmerli, 1989). These findings are surprising, given the increased resting arousal previously observed in chronically anxious patients (Lader, 1980), and they await replication. Patients with GAD did show basal elevations in muscle tension, as measured by EMG (Hoehn-Saric et al., 1989). In comparisions with patients with panic disorder, GAD patients had lower frontalis EMG levels, lower heart rates, and higher end-tidal CO_2 levels at rest (Barlow et al., 1984; Rapee, 1986). Mitral valve prolapse, a specific cardiac abnormality associated with panic disorder, does not appear to be associated with GAD (Dager, Comess, & Dunner, 1986).

On a risk-taking task, female patients with GAD were differentiable from controls only by a less pronounced skin conductance response (Hoehn-Saric et al., 1989). The authors proposed that patients with GAD may have reduced "autonomic flexibility," with a weaker autonomic response to stress and a more prolonged recovery to baseline. This would be consistent with reports of less marked skin conductance and forearm blood flow responses to stress, and slower habituation, in chronically anxious patients. Alternatively, psychophysiological differences between patients with GAD and controls may not be significant in general or may not have been elicited by the particular task used.

This raises an important methodological issue regarding biological studies of GAD. Whereas in some other anxiety disorders (e.g., specific simple phobias, post-traumatic stress disorder, social phobia, or obsessive compulsive disorder), the anxiety-provoking stimulus is known and can be applied or recreated to provoke the symptoms of the disorder, GAD is by definition a more amorphous condition, characterized by multiple unreasonable or excessive worries about situations not readily reproducible for biological studies. Thus, commonly used "stress" paradigms may or may not be stressful or provoke characteristic anxieties meaningful for individual GAD patients, whereas idiosyncrasies of the experimental environment may actually be more stressful for some subjects.

In addition, individual patients may vary in the organ system affected by anxiety. For example, GAD patients with predominant cardiac complaints showed more heart interbeat interval variability with stress than did GAD patients with few cardiac complaints (Hoehn-Saric et al., 1989). Complex interactions of type of stressful task, the types of situations or stimuli most bothersome to the individual patient, and other experimental factors may interact to yield confusing or nonsignificant results in studies using standard stress procedures in a heterogeneous population.

Sleep

In one sleep EEG study (Reynolds, Shaw, Newton, Coble, & Kupfer, 1983), patients with GAD showed more stage 2 sleep, a lower rapid eye movement (REM) percentage, longer REM latency, and less REM activity than patients with major depression. However, 6 of the 10 GAD patients in this study had additional diagnoses, including depression, schizotypal features, and substance abuse. Papadimitriou, Kerkhofs, Kempenaers, and Mendlewicz (1988) and Papadimitriou, Linkowski, Kerkhofs, Kempenaers, and Mendlewicz (1988) found increased sleep onset latency, less total sleep time, and decreased stage 2 sleep in more homogeneous groups of GAD patients. These changes differentiate patients with GAD from those with major depression, who show shorter REM latencies than anxious patients, and from those with panic disorder, who have been found to have shorter REM latency, decreased REM density, and increased movement time than do controls (Uhde et al., 1984; Dube et al., 1986).

Lactate Infusion Studies

Sodium lactate infusion, first used by Pitts and McClure (1967) in patients with anxiety neurosis (see above), provokes panic symptoms in 60–70% of patients with panic attacks, but in fewer than 10% of controls or patients without panic attacks (Liebowitz et al., 1984; Cowley & Arana, 1990). Lactate infusion induced significant anxiety, but not panic attacks, in patients with GAD without a history of panic attacks (Cowley, Dager, McClellan, Roy-Byrne, & Dunner, 1988). Patients with GAD were clearly differentiable from normal controls in their response to lactate, but were much less likely to display an abrupt, intense panic response. This study reinforces the biological and diagnostic differentiation of GAD from panic disorder.

Neurotransmitter Systems

Benzodiazepines

The most widely used pharmacological treatments for generalized anxiety have been the benzodiazepines. The recent identification of specific, high-affinity benzodiazepine-binding sites in the human brain has raised the possibility that chronic anxiety may be related to abnormalities in this receptor system (Tallman, Paul, Skolnick, & Gallagher, 1980; Braestrup & Nielson, 1982). Benzodiazepines exert their effects by binding to these specific receptor sites, which are closely associated with receptors for gamma-aminobutyric acid (GABA), the major inhibitory neurotransmitter in the mammalian brain. Benzodiazepine receptor agonists increase the frequency of openings of the chloride ionophore of the GABA receptor complex, thus enhancing the effects of GABA.

Several lines of evidence suggest that this receptor system may be involved in human anxiety. Beta-carbolines, benzodiazepine receptor inverse agonists, are anxiogenic in animals and humans (Ninan et al., 1982; Dorow, Horowski, Paschelke, Amin, & Braestrup, 1983). Alterations in number and function of benzodiazepine receptors are seen in animal models of anxiety, such as Maudsley-reactive rats (Robertson, Martin, & Candy, 1978). In animals, acute stress leads to rapid changes in the function of the chloride ionophore coupled with the central GABA–benzodiazepine receptor (Havoundjian, Paul, & Skolnick, 1986).

One study of normal humans has shown an increase in the density of peripheral benzodiazepine-binding sites in platelets in subjects undergoing an examination versus unstressed controls (Karp, Weizman, Tyano, & Gavish, 1989). This same research group has also reported decreased numbers of platelet benzodiazepine-binding sites in patients with GAD, and an up-regulation of these binding sites with chronic diazepam treatment (Weizman et al., 1987). However, these peripheral platelet benzodiazepine-binding sites are pharmacologically distinct from central benzodiazepine receptors. Unlike the central receptors, they are unassociated with the GABA–chloride ionophore complex. Thus, the significance of these results is unclear.

Recent studies from our laboratory suggest that the function of central benzodiazepine receptors may be altered in anxiety disorders. We have recently shown reduced sensitivity to diazepam (as measured by diazepam's effects in lowering catecholamine levels and slowing the velocity of saccadic eye movements) in patients with panic disorder as compared with control subjects (Roy-Byrne et al., 1989; Roy-Byrne, Cowley, Greenblatt, Shader, & Hommer, 1990). These results suggest possible decreased functional sensitivity of the benzodiazepine–GABA receptor complex in panic disorder. Preliminary results in a small group of patients with GAD suggest sub-sensitivity to diazepam in this group also; in this study, slowing of saccadic eye movements was used as the measure of diazepam effects (Roy-Byrne, Cowley, Greenblatt, Shader, & Hommer, 1991). Patients with GAD, like those with panic disorder, showed no differences from control subjects in the effects of diazepam on cortisol, ACTH, and growth hormone levels.

Interestingly, although there were no correlations in the panic disorder group between benzodiazepine sensitivity and arousal, we found significant correlations in the GAD group between the effective dose of diazepam required to reduce saccadic eye movement velocity by 30% on the one hand, and baseline cortisol and ACTH levels on the other. These preliminary data are consistent with a hypothesis that anxiety or arousal in GAD patients are closely related to the function of the benzodiazepine receptor system. These results must be replicated. However, further investigation in this area may elucidate the pathophysiology of at least some cases of GAD and help to reduce the heterogeneity of the disorder.

Serotonin

A nonbenzodiazepine anxiolytic, buspirone, which has recently been marketed and shown efficacy in the treatment of GAD, is a serotonin (5-HT; in this case, 5-HT_{1A}) receptor agonist, suggesting a possible role of serotonergic receptor systems in chronic anxiety. Animal studies suggest that increased activity of serotonergic pathways, especially the ascending dorsal raphe system, may be involved in the production of pathological anxiety (File, 1984); in humans, enhancement of serotonergic function by the 5-HT agonist m-chlorophenylpiperazine is anxiogenic (Charney, Woods, Goodman, & Heninger, 1987). The role of 5-HT in GAD has not yet been tested.

Caffeine/Adenosine

Caffeine produces anxiety and panic in both anxious patients and, to a lesser degree, control subjects, at doses theoretically lower than those required for its antagonism of benzodiazepine receptors (Charney, Heninger, & Jatlow, 1985). The anxiogenic effects of caffeine may be mediated by its antagonism of central adenosine receptors, suggesting a possible role for these receptors in the pathophysiology of chronic anxiety.

Other Neurotransmitters

Other neurotransmitters of potential significance in anxiety disorders include L-glutamic acid in its actions on N-methyl-aspartate (NMDA) receptors and corticotropin-releasing factor (CRF). Selective antagonists of the excitatory NMDA receptors have been shown in animal models to have antiepileptic, muscle relaxant, and anxiolytic properties (see Stephens, Meldrum, Weidmann, Schneider, & Grutzner, 1986).

CRF, the major physiological regulator of ACTH, is widely distributed in the brain. Preclinical studies suggest that CRF may be involved in stress responses and anxiety (reviewed in Butler & Nemeroff, 1990). CRF increases neuronal activity, secretion of epinephrine and norepinephrine from the adrenal medulla, heart rate, and blood pressure. In animals, CRF decreases exploration and contact with novel stimuli, while increasing behaviors typical of arousal or stress (e.g., locomotion, grooming, rearing, and sniffing). Central administration of CRF inhibits the normal habituation process and has anxiogenic effects in conflict models of anxiety used to test anxiolytic drugs. Acute and chronic stress results in changes in CRF concentrations in the brain, and the CRF antagonist, alpha-helical $\text{CRF}_{9\text{-}41}$, decreases stress-induced behaviors.

Cerebral Blood Flow and Metabolism

One of the most exciting recent developments in the study of the human brain is the ability to measure cerebral blood flow (CBF), oxygen consumption, and glucose metabolism. In most situations, these measures are closely related to the activity of the brain, and can thus be used to examine both global changes and regional differences in brain function accompanying a wide range of normal states as well as psychiatric disorders.

CBF and oxygen consumption were first assessed in humans by measuring differences in concentrations of oxygen and inhaled nitrous oxide between the femoral artery and internal jugular vein (Kety & Schmidt, 1948). This nitrous oxide technique yielded information regarding whole-brain blood flow and oxygen consumption, but was invasive and did not allow study of regional differences. Using this technique, Kety (1950) noted increased cerebral oxygen metabolism in a patient who experienced an anxiety attack during the procedure. In addition, epinephrine infusions increased CBF and oxygen consumption by about 20% (King, Sokoloff, & Wechsler, 1952). This was presumably a result of increased arousal and anxiety, since there were no changes in vascular resistance.

More recent measurement techniques, including xenon-133 inhalation and positron emission tomography (PET), have been used to study arousal and anxiety and allow assessment of both global and regional brain activity. In normals, increased arousal, such as that seen during REM sleep, mental tasks, and seizures, is associated with increased CBF (Mathew, Weinman, & Claghorn, 1980). Decreased arousal during drowsiness, sleep, and semicoma is associated with reduced CBF. Normal subjects in a resting, awake state show two patterns of increased CBF when presented with a stimulus or task. The first is a diffuse and general increase, which habituates with repeated exposure to the same situation; the second is a focal increase in the anatomic region corresponding to the sensory modality activated during the procedure.

Although these findings suggest a straightforward relationship between arousal on the one hand and CBF and metabolism on the other, arousal is not related in a simple way to anxiety. In normals, CBF may vary in a curvilinear fashion with anxiety level. Gur et al. (1987) found that among normal volunteers, those with lower baseline anxiety levels showed increases in CBF with increasing anxiety induced by a cognitive task. Those with higher baseline anxiety, however, showed decreased CBF with increasing anxiety. In another study by the same group (Gur et al., 1988), normals with moderate anxiety performed better and displayed greater increases in CBF than those with low or high anxiety levels.

In one study of patients with DSM-III GAD, patients displayed nonsignificant decreases in cortical blood flow compared with controls, and significant negative correlations between state anxiety and CBF in most brain regions (Mathew, Weinman, & Claghorn, 1980). In controls and patients with GAD undergoing CO_2 inhalation and patients with panic disorder given acetazolamide, there were no differences between diagnostic groups in anxiety induced by the procedures, but those subjects in all three groups who did become anxious showed significantly less of an increase in CBF with these two potent vasodilators (Mathew & Wilson, 1988, 1989). The authors postulate a vasoconstrictive factor associated with anxiety, perhaps acting via sympathetic innervation of cerebral vessels. Differences between these studies and the results of the nitrous oxide studies cited above may result from the examination of cortical blood flow with xenon-133, as opposed to whole-brain blood flow with nitrous oxide (Mathew, Weinman, & Claghorn, 1980). In addition, CBF patterns may vary with the type of anxiety (e.g., anticipatory vs. acute, psychic vs. somatic) experienced (Mathew, Weinman, & Claghorn, 1980; Zohar et al., 1989).

Regional variation in brain activity with anxiety is suggested by findings of increased right-sided glucose utilization and CBF in anxious normal volunteers (Reivich, Gur, & Alavi, 1983) and increased temporal cortex blood flow in a PET study of volunteers anticipating an electric shock (Reisman, Fusselman, Fox, & Raichle, 1989). In nonpsychiatric controls, nonsedating doses of diazepam produce decreased right-hemispheric blood flow, especially in the frontal lobe (Mathew, Wilson, & Daniel, 1985), while patients with DSM-III GAD treated with clorazepate for 21 days showed decreased right frontal and right occipital cerebral glucose metabolic rates (Buchsbaum et al., 1987).

Imaging studies are still in their infancy. Although many factors such as handedness, age, sex, and pCO_2 (i.e., degree of hyperventilation) are routinely taken into account in these carefully done studies, there remain signficant technical problems associated with the experimental setting, anxiety induced by the procedure, and interpretation of data, epecially regarding regional brain activity. Findings so far are, however, intriguing in suggesting changes with anxiety that may be regional, that may differ from those seen in nonspecific states of arousal, and that may vary with different types of anxiety.

CONCLUSION

Relatively little attention has been paid to the biology of GAD. The extensive literature on the endocrine and psychophysiological effects of acute stress in normal volunteers has been used to identify measures potentially useful in finding abnormalities in patients with chronic anxiety states. However, these measures and the nonspecific stress paradigms used in laboratory studies may detect only general changes accompanying any state of heightened arousal, rather than biological abnormalities specifically associated with, or perhaps causal in, the internally generated pathological anxiety characteristic of GAD.

Chronically anxious patients have been shown to display signs of autonomic arousal at rest. The few studies of GAD completed to date show little hyperarousal at rest, but these findings require replication. Discrepancies between studies of chronic anxiety and GAD, if substantiated, may be due to the fact that resting hyperarousal is more characteristic of patients with other anxiety disorders, such as panic disorder, who were included in early studies of chronic pathological anxiety. Alternatively, differences in baseline arousal may be affected by other factors, such as severity of illness, acute distress, or the anxiety levels of the controls used as a comparison group (Rapee, in press).

Patients with chronic anxiety show weaker changes than normals with stress procedures. Recovery to baseline values and the process of habituation with repeated stimuli may be impaired. These interesting observations are consistent with the lack of "autonomic flexibility" proposed in GAD and warrant further study. Abnormalities in the process of habituation to stressful or novel stimuli, and in the biological systems subserving this process, may prove to be important in the pathophysiology of chronic anxiety states and GAD.

Patients with GAD may have abnormalities in sympathetic nervous system or hypothalamic–pituitary–adrenal axis function, but these possibilities require further study. To date, biological studies of GAD, although not giving a consistent picture of the pathophysiology of this disorder or its relationship to chronic stress in normals, have nevertheless provided evidence that GAD is biologically distinct from panic disorder and support for the diagnostic differentiation of the two syndromes.

Promising areas for further research in this area also include the function of the central benzodiazepine–GABA receptor system, serotonergic pathways, adenosine receptors, NMDA receptors, and CRF in GAD. Further family and twin studies will clarify to what extent GAD is heritable, and cerebral imaging techniques will help to determine whether GAD is associated with changes in global or focal brain activity. Refinement of diagnostic criteria and identification of more homogeneous groups of subjects with GAD or chronic generalized anxiety may facilitate future biological studies.

REFERENCES

Abelson, J. L., Glitz, D., Cameron, O. G., Lee, M. A., Bronzo, M., & Curtis, G. C. (1991). Blunted growth hormone response to clonidine in patients with generalized anxiety disorder. *Archives of General Psychiatry, 48,* 157–162.

Ackner, B. (1956). The relationship between anxiety and the level of peripheral vasomotor activity. *Journal of Psychosomatic Research*, *1*, 21–48.

Avery, D. H., Osgood, T. B., Ishiki, D. M., Wilson, L. G., Kenny, M., & Dunner, D. L. (1985). The DST in psychiatric outpatients with generalized anxiety disorder, panic disorder, or primary affective disorder. *American Journal of Psychiatry*, *142*, 844–848.

Barlow, D. H. (1988). *Anxiety and its disorders: The nature and treatment of anxiety and panic* (pp. 172–174).

Barlow, D. H., Blanchard, E. B., Vermilyea, J. A., Vermilyea, B. B., & Di Nardo, P. A. (1986). Generalized anxiety and generalized anxiety disorder: Description and reconceptualization. *American Journal of Psychiatry*, *143*, 40–44.

Barlow, D. H., Cohen, A. S., Waddell, M. T., Vermilyea, B. B., Klosko, J. S., Blanchard, E. B., & Di Nardo, P. A. (1984). Panic and generalized anxiety disorders: Nature and treatment. *Behavior Therapy*, *15*, 431–449.

Best, J. D., & Halter, J. B. (1982). Release and clearance rates of epinephrine in man: Importance of arterial measurements. *Journal of Clinical Endocrinology and Metabolism*, *55*, 263–268.

Bliss, E. L., Migeon, C. J., Branch, C. H., & Samuels, L. T. (1956). Reaction of the adrenal cortex to emotional stress. *Psychosomatic Medicine*, *18*, 56–76.

Braestrup, C., & Nielsen, M. (1982). Neurotransmitters and CNS disease: Anxiety. *Lancet*, *ii*, 1030–1034.

Breier, A., Charney, D. S., & Heninger, G. R. (1985). The diagnostic validity of anxiety disorders and their relationships to depressive disorders. *American Journal of Psychiatry*, *142*, 787–797.

Buchsbaum, M. S., Wu, J., Haier, R., Hazlett, E., Ball, R., Katz, M., Sokolski, K., Lagunas-Solar, M., & Langer, D. H. (1987). Positron emission tomography assessment of effects of benzodiazepines on regional glucose metabolic rate in patients with anxiety disorder. *Life Sciences*, *40*, 2393–2400.

Butler, P. D., & Nemeroff, C. B. (1990). Corticotropin-releasing factor as a possible cause of comorbidity in anxiety and depressive disorders. In J. D. Maser & C. R. Cloninger (Eds.), *Comorbidity of anxiety and mood disorders*. Washington, DC: American Psychiatric Press.

Charney, D. S., Heninger, G. R., & Breier, A. (1984). Noradrenergic function in panic anxiety. *Archives of General Psychiatry*, *41*, 751–753.

Charney, D. S., Heninger, G. R., & Jatlow, P. I. (1985). Increased anxiogenic effects of caffeine in panic disorders. *Archives of General Psychiatry*, *42*, 233–243.

Charney, D. S., Woods, S. W., Goodman, W. K., & Heninger, G. R. (1987). Serotonin function in anxiety: II. Effects of the serotonin agonist MCPP in panic disorder patients and healthy subjects. *Psychopharmacology*, *92*, 14–24.

Charney, D. S., Woods, S., & Heninger, G. R. (1989). Noradrenergic function in generalized anxiety disorder: Effects of yohimbine in healthy subjects and patients with generalized anxiety disorder. *Psychiatry Research*, *27*, 173–182.

Cohen, M. E., Badal, D. W., Kilpatrick, A., Reed, E. W., & White, P. D. (1951). The high family prevalence of neurocirculatory asthenia (anxiety neurosis, effort syndrome). *American Journal of Human Genetics*, *3*, 126–158.

Cohen, M. E., Consolazio, F. C., & Johnson, R. E. (1947). Blood lactate response during moderate exercise in neurocirculatory asthenia, anxiety neurosis, or effort syndrome. *Journal of Clinical Investigation, 26,* 339–342.

Cowley, D. S., & Arana, G. W. (1990). The diagnostic utility of lactate sensitivity in panic disorder. *Archives of General Psychiatry, 47,* 277–284.

Cowley, D. S., Dager, S. R., McClellan, J., Roy-Byrne, P. P., & Dunner, D. L. (1988). Response to lactate infusion in generalized anxiety disorder. *Biological Psychiatry, 24,* 409–414.

Cowley, D. S., & Roy-Byrne, P. P. (1987). Hyperventilation and panic disorder. *American Journal of Medicine, 83,* 929–937.

Crowe, R. R., Noyes, R., Pauls, D. L., & Slymen, D. J. (1983). A family study of panic disorder. *Archives of General Psychiatry, 40,* 1065–1069.

Curtis, G., Fogel, M., McEvoy, D., & Zarate, C. (1970). Urine and plasma corticosteroids, psychological tests, and effectiveness of psychological defenses. *Journal of Psychiatric Research, 7,* 237–247.

Dager, S. R., Comess, K. A., & Dunner, D. L. (1986). Differentiation of anxious patients by two dimensional echocardiographic evaluation of the mitral valve. *American Journal of Psychiatry, 143,* 533–535.

Di Nardo, P. A., O'Brien, G. T., Barlow, D. H., Waddell, M. T., & Blancard, E. B. (1983). Reliability of DSM-III anxiety disorder categories using a new structured interview. *Archives of General Psychiatry, 40,* 1070–1074.

Dongier, M., Wittkower, E. D., Stephens-Newsham, L., & Hoffman, M. M. (1956). Psychophysiological studies in thyroid function. *Psychosomatic Medicine, 18,* 310–323.

Dorow, R., Horowski, R., Paschelke, G., Amin, M., & Braestrup, C. (1983). Severe anxiety induced by FG7142, a beta-carboline ligand for benzodiazepine receptors. *Lancet, ii,* 98–99.

Dube, S., Jones, D. A., Bell, J., Davies, A., Ross, E., & Sitaram, N. (1986). Interface of panic and depression: Clinical and sleep EEG correlates. *Psychiatry Research, 19,* 119–133.

File, S. F. (1984). The neurochemistry of anxiety. In G. D. Burrows, T. R. Norman, & B. Davies (Eds.), *Anti-anxiety agents* (pp. 13–14). Amsterdam: Elsevier.

Frankenhaeuser, M. (1979). Psychoneuroendocrine approaches to the study of emotion as related to stress and coping. In H. E. Howe, Jr. (Ed.), *Nebraska Symposium on Motivation, Vol. 27* (pp. 123–23–Lincoln: 161). Lincoln: University of Nebraska Press.

Frankenhaeuser, M., & Patkai, P. (1965). Interindividual differences in catecholamine excretion during stress. *Scandinavian Journal of Psychology, 6,* 117–123.

Frosman, L. (1980). Habitual catecholamine excretion and its relation to habitual distress. *Biological Psychology, 11,* 83–97.

Gottschalk, L. A., Cleghorn, J. M., Gleser, G. C., & Iacono, J. M. (1965). Studies of relationships of emotions to plasma lipids. *Psychosomatic Medicine, 27,* 102–111.

Gur, R. C., Gur, R. E., Resnick, S. M., Skolnick, B. E., Alavi, A., & Reivich, M. (1987). The effect of anxiety on cortical cerebral blood flow and metabolism.

Journal of Cerebral Blood Flow and Metabolism, 7, 173–177.

Gur, R. C., Gur, R. E., Skolnick, B. E., Resnick, S. M., Silver, F. L., Chawluk, J., Muenz, L., Obrist, W. D., & Reivich, M. (1988). Effects of task difficulty on regional cerebral blood flow: Relationships with anxiety and performance. *Psychophysiology, 25*, 392–399.

Hardonk, H., & Beumer, H. (1979). Hyperventilation syndrome. In P. Vinken & G. Bruyn (Eds.), *Handbook of clinical neurology, Vol. 4* (pp. 309–360). New York: North-Holland.

Havoundjian, H., Paul, S. M., & Skolnick, P. (1986). Rapid, stress-induced modification of the benzodiazepine receptor-coupled chloride ionophore. *Brain Research, 375*, 401–406.

Hoehn-Saric, R., & Masek, B. J. (1981). Effects of naloxone in normals and chronically anxious patients. *Biological Psychiatry, 16*, 1041–1050.

Hoehn-Saric, R., & McLeod, D. (1988). The peripheral sympathetic nervous system: Its role in normal and pathologic anxiety. *Psychiatric Clinics of North America, 11*, 375–386.

Hoehn-Saric, R., McLeod, D. R., & Zimmerli, W. D. (1989). Somatic manifestations in women with generalized anxiety disorder: Psychophysiological responses to psychological stress. *Archives of General Psychiatry, 46*, 1113–1119.

Holmgren, A., & Strom, G. (1959). Blood lactate concentration in relation to absolute and relative work load in normal men, and in mitral stenosis, atrial septal defect and vasoregulatory asthenia. *Acta Medica Scandinavica, 163*, 185–193.

Jones, M., & Mellersh, V. (1946). A comparison of the exercise response in anxiety states and normal controls. *Psychosomatic Medicine, 8*, 180–187.

Karp, L., Weizman, A., Tyano, S., & Gavish, M. (1989). Examination stress, platelet peripheral benzodiazepine binding sites, and plasma hormone levels. *Life Sciences, 44*, 1077–1082.

Kathol, R. G., Turner, R., & Delahunt, J. (1986). Depression and anxiety associated with hyperthyroidism: Response to antithyroid therapy. *Psychosomatics, 27*, 501–505.

Kelly, D., Brown, C. C., & Shaffer, J. W. (1970). A comparison of physiological and psychological measurements of anxious patients and normal controls. *Psychophysiology, 6*, 429–441.

Kerr, W., Dalton, J., & Gliebe, P. (1937). Some physical phenomena associated with the anxiety states and their relation to hyperventilation. *Annals of Internal Medicine, 11*, 961–992.

Kety, S. S. (1950). Circulation and metabolism of the human brain in health and disease. *American Journal of Medicine, 8*, 205–217.

Kety, S. S., & Schmidt, C. F. (1948). The nitrous oxide method for the quantitative determination of cerebral blood flow in man: Theory, procedure, and normal values. *Journal of Clinical Investigation, 27*, 476–483.

Khan, A., Lee, E., Dager, S., Hyde, T., Raisys, V., Avery, D., & Dunner, D. (1986). Platelet MAO-B activity in anxiety and depression. *Biological Psychiatry, 21*, 847–849.

King, B. D., Sokoloff, L., & Wechsler, R. L. (1952). The effect of L-epinephrine and L-norepinephrine upon cerebral circulation and metabolism in man. *Journal of Clinical Investigation, 31*, 273–279.

Lader, M. H. (1967). Palmar skin conductance meaures in anxiety and phobic states. *Journal of Psychosomatic Research, 11*, 271–281.

Lader, M. H. (1980). Psychophysiological studies in anxiety. In G. Burrows & B. Davies (Eds.), *Handbook of studies on anxiety* (pp. 59–88). Amsterdam: Elsevier/North-Holland.

Lader, M. H., Gelder, M. G., & Marks, I. M. (1967). Palmar skin conductance measures as predictors of response to desensitization. *Journal of Psychosomatic Research, 11*, 283–290.

Lader, M. H., & Wing, L. (1964). Habituation of the psycho-galvanic reflex in patients with anxiety states and in normal subjects. *Journal of Neurology, Neurosurgery and Psychiatry, 27*, 210–218.

Lewis, B. (1954). Chronic hyperventilation syndrome. *Journal of the American Medical Association, 155*, 1204–1208.

Liebowitz, M. R., Feyer, A. J., Gorman, J. M., Dillon, D., Appleby, I. L., Levy, G., Anderson, S., Levitt, M., Palij, M., Davies, S. O., & Klein, D. F. (1984). Lactate provocation of panic attacks: I. Clinical and behavioral findings. *Archives of General Psychiatry, 41*, 764–770.

Malmo, R. B., Shagass, C., & Heslam, R. M. (1951). Blood pressure response to repeated brief stress in psychoneurosis: A study on adaptation. *Canadian Journal of Psychology, 5*, 167–179.

Mathew, R. J., Ho, B. T., Francis, D. J., Taylor, D. L., & Weinman, M. L. (1982). Catecholamines and anxiety. *Acta Psychiatrica Scandinavica, 65*, 142–147.

Mathew, R. J., Ho, B. T., Kralik, P., & Claghorn, J. L. (1979). Anxiety and serum prolactin. *American Journal of Psychiatry, 136*, 716–717.

Mathew, R. J., Ho, B. T., Kralik, P., Taylor, D., Semchuk, K., Weinman, M., & Claghorn, J. L. (1980). Catechol-O-methyltransferase and catecholamines in anxiety and relaxation. *Psychiatry Research, 3*, 85–91.

Mathew, R. J., Ho, B. T., Kralik, P., Weinman, M., & Claghorn, J. L. (1981). Anxiety and platelet MAO levels after relaxation training. *American Journal of Psychiatry, 138*, 371–373.

Mathew, R. J., Ho, B. T., Taylor, D. L., & Semchuk, K. M. (1981). Catecholamine and dopamine-beta-hydroxylase in anxiety. *Journal of Psychosomatic Research, 25*, 499–504.

Mathew, R. J., Weinman, M. L., & Claghorn, J. L. (1980). Anxiety and cerebral blood flow. In R. J. Mathew (Ed.), *The biology of anxiety* (pp. 23–33). New York: Brunner/Mazel.

Mathew, R. J., & Wilson, W. H. (1988). Cerebral blood flow changes induced by CO_2 in anxiety. *Psychiatry Research, 23*, 285–294.

Mathew, R. J., & Wilson, W. H. (1989). Cerebral blood flow responses to CO_2 and acetazolamide: The effect of anxiety. *Psychiatry Research, 28*, 241–242.

Mathew, R. J., Wilson, W. H., & Daniel, D. G. (1985). The effect of nonsedating doses of diazepam on regional cerebral blood flow. *Biological Psychiatry, 20*, 1109–1116.

Miyabo, S., Hisada, T., Asato, T., Mizushima, N., & Ueno, K. (1976). Growth hormone and cortisol responses to psychological stress: Comparison of normal and neurotic subjects. *Journal of Clinical Endocrinology and Metabolism, 42,* 1158–1162.

Munjack, D. J., Baltazar, P. L., DeQuattro, V., Sobin, P., Palmer, R., Zulueta, A., Crocker, B., Usigli, R., Buckwalter, G., & Leonard, M. (1990). Generalized anxiety disorder: Some biochemical aspects. *Psychiatry Research, 32,* 35–43.

Munjack, D. J., & Palmer, R. (1988). Thyroid hormones in panic disorder, panic disorder with agoraphobia, and generalized anxiety disorder. *Journal of Clinical Psychiatry, 49,* 229–231.

Nelson, G. N., Masuda, M., & Holmes, T. H. (1966). Correlation of behavior and catecholamine metabolite excretion. *Psychosomatic Medicine, 28,* 216–226.

Ninan, P. T., Insel, T. M., Cohen, R. M., Cook, J. M., Skolnick, P., & Paul, S. M. (1982). Benzodiazepine receptor-mediated experimental "anxiety" in primates. *Science, 218,* 1332–1334.

Noyes, R., Clarkson, C., Crowe, R. R., Yates, W. R., & McChesney, C. M. (1987). A family study of generalized anxiety disorder. *American Journal of Psychiatry, 144,* 1019–1024.

Papadimitriou, G. N., Kerkhofs, M., Kempenaers, C., & Mendlewicz, J. (1988). EEG sleep studies in patients with generalized anxiety disorder. *Psychiatry Research, 26,* 183–190.

Papadimitriou, G. N., Linkowski, P., Kerkhofs, M., Kempenaers, C., & Mendlewicz, J. (1988). Sleep EEG recordings in generalized anxiety disorder with significant depression. *Journal of Affective Disorders, 15,* 113–118.

Persky, H. (1957). Adrenal cortical function in anxious human subjects. Effect of corticotrophin (ACTH) on plasma hydrocortisone level and urinary hydroxycorticoid excretion. *Archives of Neurology and Psychiatry, 78,* 95–100.

Persky, H., Grinker, R. R., Hamburg, D. A., Sabshin, M. A., Korchin, S. J., Basowitz, H., & Chevalier, J. A. (1956). Adrenal cortical function in anxious human subjects. *Archives of Neurology and Psychiatry, 76,* 549–558.

Pitts, F. N., & McClure, J. N. (1967). Lactate metabolism in anxiety neurosis. *New England Journal of Medicine, 227,* 1329–1336.

Rapee, R. M. (1986). Differential response to hyperventilation in panic disorder and generalized anxiety disorder. *Journal of Abnormal Psychology, 95,* 24–28.

Rapee, R. M. (in press). Generalized anxiety disorder: A review of clinical features and theoretical concepts. *Clinical Psychology Review.*

Reiman, E. M., Fusselman, M. J., Fox, P. T., & Raichle, M. E. (1989). Neuroanatomical correlates of anticipatory anxiety. *Science, 243,* 1071–1074.

Reiss, M., Hemphill, R. E., Maggs, R., Smith, S., Haigh, C. P., & Reiss, J. M. (1951). Thyroid activity in mental patients: Evaluation by radioactive tracer methods. *British Medical Journal, i,* 1181–1183.

Reivich, M., Gur, R. C., & Alavi, A. (1983). Positron emission tomography studies of sensory stimuli, cognitive processes and anxiety. *Human Neurobiology, 2,* 25–33.

Reynolds, C. F., Shaw, D. H., Newton, T. F., Coble, P. A., & Kupfer, D. J. (1983). EEG sleep in outpatients with generalized anxiety: A preliminary comparison with depressed outpatients. *Psychiatry Research, 8,* 81–89.

Robertson, H. A., Martin, I. L., & Candy, J. M. (1978). Differences in benzodiazepine receptor binding in Maudsley reactive and Maudsley nonreactive rats. *European Journal of Pharmacology, 50,* 455–457.

Rose, R. M. (1984). Overview of endocrinology of stress. In G. M. Brown (Ed.), *Neuroendocrinology and psychiatric disorders* (pp. 95–122). New York: Raven Press.

Rosenbaum, A. H., Schatzberg, A. F., Jost, F. A., Cross, P. D., Wells, L. A., Jiang, N. S., & Maruta, T. (1983). Urinary free cortisol levels in anxiety. *Psychosomatic, 24,* 835–837.

Roy-Byrne, P. P., & Cowley, D. S. (1988). Biological aspects of panic disorder. *Psychiatric Annals, 18,* 457–463.

Roy-Byrne, P. P., Cowley, D. S., Greenblatt, D. J., Shader, R. I., & Hommer, D. (1990). Reduced benzodiazepine sensitivity in panic disorder. *Archives of General Psychiatry, 47,* 534–538.

Roy-Byrne, P. P, Cowley, D S., Greenblatt, D. J., Shader, R. I., & Hommer, D. (1991). *Benzodiazepine sensitivity in generalized anxiety disorder.* Unpublished manuscript.

.Roy-Byrne, P. P., Lewis, N., Villacres, E., Diem, H., Greenblatt, D. J., Shader, R. I., & Veith, R. C. (1989). Preliminary evidence of benzodiazepine sub-sensitivity in panic disorder. *Biological Psychiatry, 26,* 744–748.

Rubin, L. S. (1964). Autonomic dysfunction as a concomitant of neurotic behavior. *Journal of Nervous and Mental Disease, 138,* 558–574.

Schweizer, E. E., Swenson, D. M., Winokur, A., Rickels, K., & Maislin, G. (1986). The dexamethasone suppression test in generalised anxiety disorder. *British Journal of Psychiatry, 149,* 320–322.

Sevy, S., Papadimitriou, G. M., Surmont, D. W., Goldman, S., & Mendlewicz, J. (1989). Noradrenergic function in generalized anxiety disorder, major depressive disorder, and healthy subjects. *Biological Psychiatry, 25,* 141–152.

Sokoloff, L., Mangold, R., Wechsler, R. L., Kennedy, C., & Kety, S. S. (1955). The effect of mental arithmetic on cerebral circulation and metabolism. *Journal of Clinical Investigation, 34,* 1101–1108.

Stephens, D. N., Meldrum, B. S., Weidmann, R., Schneider, C., & Grutzner, M. (1986). Does the excitatory amino acid receptor antagonist 2-APH exhibit anxiolytic activity? *Psychopharmacology, 90,* 166–169.

Suess, W., Alexander, A., Smith, D., Sweeney, H., & Marion, J. (1980). The effects of psychological stress on respiration: A preliminary study of anxiety and the hyperventilation syndrome. *Psychophysiology, 17,* 535–540.

Tallman, J. F., Paul, S. M., Skolnick, P., & Gallagher, D. W. (1980). Receptors for the age of anxiety: Pharmacology of the benzodiazepines. *Science, 207,* 274–281.

Tiller, J. W. G., Biddle, N., Maguire, K. P., & Davies, B. M. (1988). The dexamethasone suppression test and plasma dexamethasone in generalized anxiety disorder. *Biological Psychiatry, 23,* 261–270.

Torgerson, S. (1983). Genetic factors in anxiety disorders. *Archives of General Psychiatry, 40,* 1085–1089.

Tyrer, P. (1985). Neurosis divisible? *Lancet, i,* 685–688.

Uhde, T. W., Roy-Byrne, P. P., Gillin, J. C., Mendelson, W. B., Boulenger, J. P., Vittone, B. J., & Post, R. M. (1984). The sleep of patients with panic disorder: A preliminary report. *Psychiatry Research, 12,* 251–259.

Weizman, R., Tanne, Z., Granek, M., Karp, L., Golomb, M., Tyano, S., & Gavish, M. (1987). Peripheral benzodiazepine binding sites on platelet membranes are increased during diazepam treatment of anxious patients. *European Journal of Pharmacology, 138,* 289–292.

Wheeler, E. O., White, P. D., Reed, E., & Cohen, M. E. (1948). Familial incidence of neurocirculatory asthenia ("anxiety neurosis," "effort syndrome"). *Journal of Clinical Investigation, 27,* 562.

Wyatt, R. J., Porkorny, B., Kupfer, D. J., Snyder, F., & Engelman, K. (1971). Resting plasma catecholamine concentrations in patients with depression and anxiety. *Archives of General Psychiatry, 24,* 65–70.

Zohar, J., Insel, T. R., Berman, K. F., Foa, E. B., Hill, J. L., & Weinberger, D. R. (1989). Anxiety and cerebral blood flow during behavioral challenge. *Archives of General Psychiatry, 46,* 505–510.

4

Psychological Factors Involved in Generalized Anxiety

RONALD M. RAPEE
University of Queensland

The importance of trait anxiety for the manifestation of a wide variety of behaviors, as well as its influence on many behaviors, has been recognized for years; by contrast, chronic anxiety as a problem in its own right has received far less attention. Thus, for example, we have known about the effects of anxiety on performance since the early years of this century (Yerkes & Dodson, 1908). Similarly, the importance of trait anxiety as a motivator for learning certain relationships has received considerable attention (Taylor, 1951). However, the development and maintenance of a general tendency to be anxious (chronic, trait, or generalized anxiety [GA]), at least from a psychological perspective, has rarely been directly investigated.

This deficit has begun to change over the last few years, perhaps partly due to the influence of the *Diagnostic and Statistical Manual of Mental Disorders*, third edition (DSM-III; American Psychiatric Association, 1980). In 1980 the DSM-III introduced the category of generalized anxiety disorder (GAD) to refer to individuals who experienced chronic, heightened levels of diffuse anxiety and did not meet criteria for any other anxiety disorder, such as panic disorder or phobias. Although such anxiety states had been described before under the label of "free-floating anxiety" (Wolpe, 1958) or "anxiety neurosis" (Marks & Lader, 1973), this was the first widely accepted indication that such a disorder existed as a significant problem for a number of individuals. With the removal of GAD from "wastebasket" status in the DSM-III-R (American Psychiatric Association, 1987), this disorder has taken on even more importance. In addition, the DSM-III-

R has defined worry as one of the major features in GAD, strongly emphasizing a psychological focus to the disorder.

Studies investigating the nature of GAD have indicated that GA can be identified as a construct that is distinct from other forms of anxiety, such as panic attacks (Beck, Laude, & Bohnert, 1974; Hibbert, 1984; Rapee, 1985). It is unfortunate, therefore, that much of what is currently known about the nature of GAD has come from studies in which GAD is not the main topic of interest, but rather is included as a comparison condition to other anxiety disorders (Rapee, in press). Greater understanding of the nature, development, and maintenance of GAD is likely to improve treatment options (see Chapter 10, this volume), as well as being of interest in its own right. Although research into the psychological factors underlying GA is still in its infancy, some promising developments have emerged in recent years. This chapter reviews this literature and attempts to place it into a cohesive framework.

GENERALIZED ANXIETY VERSUS GENERALIZED ANXIETY DISORDER

Before the chapter launches into a discussion of etiological and maintaining factors, it is important to define the constructs of interest. In the present context, the main distinction requiring clarification is that between GA and GAD.

GA is a trait construct that can be identified in all individuals to a greater or lesser degree. The focus in the present chapter is on high levels of GA, but these are not necessarily only applicable to GAD. They are likely to be found across all of the anxiety disorders (Barlow, Blanchard, Vermilyea, Vermilyea, & Di Nardo, 1986), and probably in many other psychological disorders as well.

GAD, on the other hand, refers to a specific constellation of symptoms as defined in the DSM-III-R. The degree of overlap between GA and GAD is open to empirical investigation, but it is likely to be large; in fact, GAD can be seen as a disorder of relatively pure, high GA (Rapee, in press). Nevertheless, some additional characteristics are presumably required for a high level of a given trait to become a disorder. Thus, it is important at some levels to continue to distinguish between these constructs.

In the present chapter, the terms GA and GAD are used precisely to refer to the respective definitions given here. Much of the chapter focuses on GA, because of the relative lack of research specifically targeting GAD. However, given the large overlap, it is assumed that many of the psychological factors important in GA are equally applicable to GAD.

FACTORS ASSOCIATED WITH ONSET

Studies investigating the onset or etiology of GAD have been conspicuously absent. This is not especially surprising, given the fact that GAD is a long-term disorder, with many studies indicating an age of onset as far back as an individual can remember (Barlow et al., 1986; Rapee, 1985). Thus, some would suggest that GAD could be conceptualized as a characterological disorder (Rapee, in press; see also Chapter 6, this volume), making investigation of its onset extremely difficult.

In line with such a trait conceptualization of GAD, three studies have retrospectively examined childhood factors in this disorder, although all three have suffered from methodological problems. Hoehn-Saric (1981) compared two groups of GAD patients, one with and one without panic attacks, on the Childhood Behavior Disturbance Scale (a measure of minimal brain dysfunction symptoms). The theoretical purpose of using this measure was not made clear, and no differences were found between groups.

Raskin, Peeke, Dickman, and Pinsker (1982) used semistructured interviews to compare 17 panic disorder subjects with 16 GAD subjects on a number of childhood and familial factors, including parental history of anxiety; history of familial psychiatric disorders; and presence of early separations, childhood abuse, childhood separation disorder, or a "grossly disturbed childhood environment." The GAD subjects did not score higher than the panic disorder subjects on any measures and reported a less "grossly disturbed childhood environment."

Finally, Torgerson (1986) compared 32 GAD patients with 29 panic disorder patients on a number of childhood factors, including nightmares, various fears, free-floating anxiety, depression, parental divorce, separation from parents, enuresis, stomach pains, and headaches. There were no significant differences between groups, except that the panic disorder patients reported more chronic anxiety in childhood.

Clearly, the question of early childhood influences on the development of GAD remains wide open. As already noted, the studies discussed above had a number of methodological flaws, including the lack of a normal control group. Given the fact that panic disorder subjects are likely to have high levels of GA (Barlow et al., 1986), the lack of differences between groups is hardly surprising. In addition, none of the studies appeared to have a strong theoretical base, and this is needed in any future investigation.

One interesting animal study deserves mention, since it may have implications for the development of GA and thus for that of GAD. Mineka, Gunnar, and Champoux (1986) reared two groups of monkeys in environments differing in the amount of available control over appetitive events. The "master" group had available various manipulanda that would result in presentation of reinforcements, contingent upon the appropriate response. The "yoked" group received the same rewards contingent upon the master group's responses. A variety of behavioral tests indicated that the master group displayed more exploratory behavior, less fearful responses, and more coping responses to social separation than the yoked controls. These results indicate the likely importance of early experience with controllability in the later development of nonfearful behavior.

FACTORS ASSOCIATED WITH MAINTENANCE

Although there have been relatively few empirical investigations of maintaining factors in GAD, a number of authors have discussed theoretical aspects of chronic anxiety. These theories have focused primarily on the importance of two fundamental constructs: threat and control. Some authors identify essentially one or the other of these constructs as basic to the manifestation of chronic anxiety; most acknowledge the importance of both, but tend to focus on one or the other.

Mathews and MacLeod (1987) describe an information-processing model of clinical anxiety, which focuses on perceived threat as the central feature. According to these authors, anxiety is maintained by a tendency to pay excessive attention to possible threat, to assign the most threatening interpretations possible to events, and to be especially efficient at acquiring threatening information. This model is based on an innovative series of empirical investigations, many of which are described below.

The fundamental aspects of this model are derived from Beck's theory of anxiety (e.g., Beck, Emery, & Greenberg, 1985). According to these authors, anxiety is a response to perceived danger. Chronic or pathological anxiety occurs in individuals who consistently misperceive danger because of distortions in the way they process information. Such individuals are characterized by cognitive schemas biased toward the selective processing of information related to personal threat. Although Beck et al. (1985) appear to emphasize threat as a major construct underlying anxiety disorders, they also point to the importance of perceptions of control. Specifically, they use Lazarus's (1966) notion of secondary appraisal to suggest that anxiety is also mediated by perceptions of an individual's resources for controlling the threat. Presumably, individuals high in GA would have a general tendency toward low perceptions of available control resources, though this is not made clear.

In a similar fashion, two early theories of chronic anxiety (Lader, 1972; Spielberger, 1972) also emphasize the importance of perceived threat, but acknowledge a mediating role for personal control or coping skills. Lader (1972) suggests that pathological trait anxiety involves an excessive tendency to appraise events as threatening, and that this threat appraisal is influenced by the individual's coping mechanisms. Similarly, Spielberger (1972) suggests that individuals high in trait anxiety are more likely to perceive events as threatening. However, following threat appraisal, state anxiety can be quickly reduced by effective coping responses.

A much stronger emphasis on perceived control in anxiety is presented by Barlow (1988; see also Chapter 1, this volume). Barlow's theory is somewhat different from the others discussed here, since he postulates a fundamental difference between fear and anxiety. Fear is a basic emotion precipitated by real or unreal danger, whereas anxiety is viewed as a cognitive–affective construct mediated primarily by low perceptions of personal control. According to Barlow, GAD is essentially a disorder of anxiety, and such individuals are characterized by a strong sense of loss of control over crucial internal and external events.

From these models of chronic anxiety, it is clear that to a greater or lesser degree, two basic constructs have been implicated in the maintenance of GA: perceptions of personal threat, and a low perceived control. In addition, some of the theorists have emphasized the importance of biased perceptions and interpretations demonstrated by individuals with anxiety disorders. These features, and much of the empirical research that has been conducted in this area, can be clearly described by means of an information-processing model. Thus, such a model is now presented and used as a basis for discussing the scant empirical literature.

AN INFORMATION-PROCESSING MODEL OF GENERALIZED ANXIETY

There has been a recent trend in research on the anxiety disorders, following similar earlier trends in depression and schizophrenia research, to focus on aspects of the way in which anxious subjects process information. Although this orientation is still relatively new in its application to anxiety, there currently exist enough empirical data that it is possible to begin to summarize some of the more obvious information-processing aspects of GA. The remainder of this chapter presents some of these theoretical concepts and examines their empirical support. Doing this should make many of the limitations of this research and future requirements more apparent.

The term "information processing" covers a broad range of functions and processes. Thus, it is difficult to discuss a single, comprehensive schematic model. Rather, four broad areas of information processing that appear to have relevance for GA are discussed separately: attentional resources, long-term memory, working memory, and self-schemas.

Attentional Resources

The first stage in the model suggests that individuals with high levels of GA allocate attentional resources preferentially to threatening stimuli. This differential allocation may have one or both of two broad effects. First, it is predicted that some resources will be continuously allocated to detect the presence of threat in the environment as efficiently as possible. Therefore, when threatening stimuli exist in the environment, individuals high in GA should be more likely to detect them and should detect them sooner than nonanxious subjects should. Second, it may be predicted that when threat is detected, individuals high in GA will focus more of their attentional resources on the threat than will nonanxious subjects. Thus, for example, in the face of equivalent threat, those high in GA should have greater difficulty performing a secondary, attention-demanding task than should those low in GA.

Of course, individuals high in GA (and thus those with GAD) experience higher levels of general arousal than do nonanxious individuals (Fridlund, Hatfield, Cottam, & Fowler, 1986; Mathew, Ho, Kralick, Taylor, & Claghorn, 1981). Thus, not only will the direction of attentional allocation differ, but there will also be a difference in the form of the attentional focus. More specifically, attention and arousal interact in such a way that greater arousal results in a reduced breadth of focus (Easterbrook, 1959) and possibly also a greater variability (Eysenck & Mathews, 1987). In addition, there is some suggestion that increased arousal results in a greater number of attentional resources' being available for utilization (Kahneman, 1973). Although these effects must be kept in mind when examining the literature on attention in GA (since they may have influenced some of the results), they are not discussed at great length here, because they are probably more important for explaining performance effects than for explaining the maintenance of GA.

The majority of the research has focused on the issue of whether subjects high in GA are more efficient at detecting threat in the environment, and most empirical evidence seems to support this hypothesis. Mathews and colleagues have conducted three studies, using slightly different methodologies, which have all shown an attentional bias toward threatening stimuli in high-GA and GAD subjects (MacLeod, Mathews, & Tata, 1986; Mathews & MacLeod, 1985, 1986). In the first of these studies (Mathews & MacLeod, 1985), the authors presented a modified version of the Stroop (1935) color-naming task to GA subjects and nonanxious controls. The anxious subjects were slower to color-name threat-related words than neutral words, whereas the nonanxious controls were equal in color-naming time for both lists. These results imply that extra processing resources were allocated to the threat-related words by the GA subjects, thus interfering with their performance of the task. Because other emotional words were not included, the study is open to the criticism that anxious subjects may simply be more responsive to any emotional word (Martin, Williams, & Clark, 1988). However, there was some evidence in the study that GA subjects who reported more concern over physical cues responded specifically to the words related to physical threat, and not those related to social threat. Similar specificity effects have been demonstrated in a comparison of subjects with social phobia and panic disorder (Hope, Rapee, Heimberg, & Dombeck, 1990).

The finding of an attentional bias toward threat in GA subjects was replicated in two later studies, using a dot probe detection task (MacLeod et al., 1986) and a dichotic listening task (Mathews & MacLeod, 1986). Once again, the studies indicated that anxious subjects allocate more attentional resources to threat words. In addition, all studies indicated that this attentional allocation seems to occur at an unconscious or unaware level, since recognition tasks did not demonstrate that subjects recognized any words at an above-chance level. Furthermore, in the dichotic listening task, a subgroup of subjects was interrupted during the task; these subjects were unable to repeat the word that had just been presented on the unattended channel.

One of the major issues not addressed in the above-described studies is the degree to which this attentional allocation is a consistent characteristic of the individual. All of these studies compared anxious and nonanxious subjects, who differed not only in trait anxiety but also in state anxiety. In fact, in the Stroop study (Mathews & MacLeod, 1985), state anxiety was found to correlate more strongly with interference than trait anxiety.

In an attempt to address this question, MacLeod and Mathews (1988) tested subjects high and low in trait anxiety, using a dot probe detection task at two times: once 12 weeks before an examination, and again 1 week before the examination. The results indicated that state anxiety interacted with trait anxiety: Only the subjects high in trait anxiety showed an increased allocation of attention 1 week before the exam. In addition, this effect only occurred with words related to social-evaluative threat (i.e., related to the exam) and not with words related to physical threat. There was a slight tendency for low-anxiety subjects to focus attention away from exam-related words on the second occasion. These findings are consistent with those of a questionnaire study by Butler and Mathews (1987): Subjects increased their prediction of risk as they approached an exam (increased state anxiety), but only for exam-related threat.

One other study has examined the state–trait question in relation to attention (Broadbent & Broadbent, 1988). These authors utilized the dot probe paradigm used by MacLeod et al. (1986) with nonclinical subjects, and replicated the finding that subjects with greater levels of anxiety focused more attention on threat-related words. The most consistent relationship between anxiety and attention to threat was found with trait anxiety. State anxiety demonstrated an inconsistent effect, showing a relationship in one experiment but not in three others. Thus, Broadbent and Broadbent have suggested that the tendency to orient toward threat is a general characteristic of the individual, rather than a temporary feature of being anxious at a particular time.

The issue of whether subjects with GAD actually allocate more attentional resources to stimuli than nonanxious subjects when both are faced with objective threat has not been investigated. Once threat is detected, it is likely that both anxious and nonanxious subjects will allocate some resources to monitoring of the threat. The question of whether anxious subjects allocate more attention to the threat is open for empirical investigation.

Long-Term Memory

Hypotheses about the structure of long-term memory in GA have been primarily based on clinical insight with GAD patients, much of which has been described above. As mentioned earlier, Beck et al. (1985) see chronically anxious individuals as characterized by highly active threat schemas. Thus, it is suggested that information related to threat is more easily accessed by anxious subjects. This greater availability of threat-related information should in turn influence subjects' estimates of risk—a suggestion that has received some empirical support (Butler & Mathews, 1983). Importantly, given the generalized focus of GAD patients' concerns, such individuals would presumably be characterized by strong associations between a broad range of stimuli and threats (Rapee, in press).

A second area suggested to be involved in anxiety (described above) is a lack of perceived control (see Barlow, 1988, and Chapter 1, this volume). According to Barlow, individuals with GAD are characterized by general perceptions of uncontrollability over events. Thus, putting these two concepts together, one could suggest that the experience of anxiety depends on the perception of a stimulus associated with threat *and* a belief that one has no control over that stimulus. Anxiety should not occur if either the stimulus is not associated with threat or the stimulus is associated with complete potential control. A schematic representation of this relationship in long-term memory is shown in Figure 4.1. In this diagram, the affect of anxiety is represented as a distinct information node in memory,

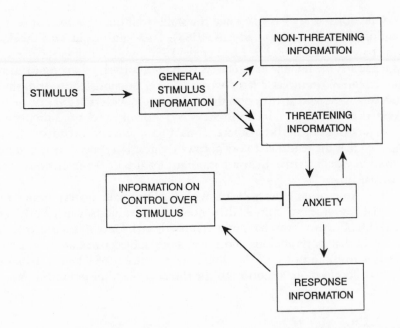

FIGURE 4.1. An information-processing model of the maintenance of GAD. From "Generalized Anxiety Disorder: A Review of Clinical Features and Theoretical Concepts" by R. M. Rapee, in press. *Clinical Psychology Review, 11.* Copyright 1991 by Pergamon Press. Reprinted by permission.

consistent with a conceptualization by Bower (1981). Information related to threat has a positive association with anxiety, whereas information related to control has an inhibitory association with anxiety. There is also a loop between threat-related information and anxiety, representing the hypothesized influence of current or state anxiety on specific threat-related information. In other words, as the anxiety node is accessed, it in turn will make the threat-related information that triggered it even more accessible. Three sources of evidence are required to support this model: (1) evidence on the easy accessibility of threat-related information; (2) evidence on the interaction between current anxiety levels and threat; and (3) evidence on the easy accessibility of information related to lack of control.

By far the strongest evidence exists to support the suggestion that GA is associated with a lowered threshold for threat-related information. This evidence has taken two broad forms: the tendency for GAD patients to respond with interpretations of threat when presented with ambiguous stimuli, and the ability of GAD patients to retrieve threat-related information after being presented with it.

In an early study, Butler and Mathews (1983) presented a series of ambiguous scenarios to subjects and asked them to indicate the thought in which they would be most likely to engage in each situation. Subjects high in GA were more likely to indicate a threatening intepretation than nonanxious controls were. Subjects were also asked to rate the likelihood that various events (both positive and negative) would occur in their own lives. Given that subjective probability estimates are suggested to be based on the ease with which specific outcomes come to mind (Tversky & Kahneman, 1974), higher probability ratings for threatening events would indicate greater accessibility of threat-related information. The results indicated that subjects high in GA did rate the probability of personally experiencing threatening events as higher than did nonanxious controls. There was no difference for positive events. Thes data were replicated in a later study, using students high and low in trait anxiety (Butler & Mathews, 1987).

Using a different methodology, Mathews, Richards, and Eysenck (1989) presented a series of homophones to subjects with GAD and non-anxious controls, and asked them to write down the words they heard. Each word had one of two possible spellings: a neutral spelling (e.g., "dye") or a threat-related spelling (e.g., "die"). GADs were more likely to use the threat-related spelling of homophones than were controls, indicating greater accessing of threat-linked information in the former group.

The second form of evidence for a lowered threshold for threat-related information in high GA has been obtained through memory studies. One of the probable functions of schemas is to aid encoding (Brewer & Nakamura, 1984). Thus, if subjects high in GA have highly elaborated and efficient threat schemas, they should encode threat-related information more efficiently than other individuals, and in turn should be better able to access this encoded material. Unfortunately, the few memory studies conducted to date have been somewhat inconsistent.

In one such study, subjects were asked to rate a larger number of words on their applicability to either themselves or a television personality. They were then unexpectedly given a recall task followed by a recognition task (Mogg, Mathews, & Weinman, 1987). Surprisingly, GAD subjects did not remember more threat words than nonanxious controls did. In fact, there was a trend for nonanxious subjects to recall more threat-related words than did the GAD subjects, and there was a significant effect in the same direction on the recognition task. The authors suggested that although individuals with GAD may still encode threat-related information more efficiently, they may avoid extensive elaboration of the information as a secondary response, which may inhibit retrieval. However, it is possible that a longer delay between word presentation and retrieval might have produced different results (Rapee, in press), since schema-consistent retrieval effects often only emerge with time (Brewer & Nakamura, 1984).

In a later study, an attempt was made to differentiate between implicit memory (basically automatic and nonconscious) and explicit memory (controlled, conscious) in anxiety (Mathews, Mogg, May, & Eysenck, 1989). More efficient encoding of threat information in GAD subjects should show up in an implicit memory task, despite any secondary avoidance. Indeed, the results showed a significant difference between the GAD and control subjects on a word completion task (implicit memory), but not on a cued recall task (explicit memory). However, the results were somewhat confusing, since there was a significant correlation between trait anxiety and recall but not between trait anxiety and word completion.

Thus, support for the hypothesis that individuals high in GA have extensively elaborated threat schemas and a lowered threshold for threat-related information is supported by studies examining the availability of threat-linked information in an ambiguous situation. However, the question of more efficient encoding of such information has provided confusing data in memory studies and requires further investigation.

The question of the interaction between current anxiety levels and threat has received far less attention. Most studies discussed to date have compared GAD subjects with nonanxious controls (or recovered patients), and have thus simultaneously manipulated state and trait anxiety. It is generally assumed that the effects are largely due to trait anxiety, and indeed stronger correlations are generally found with trait anxiety than with state anxiety. However, specific manipulations of one while keeping the other steady are exceptional. The likely interaction between state anxiety and internal representations of threat is suggested by evidence that current mood often influences information processing (Bower, 1981). More recent reviews have suggested that this is especially so for encoding of information; the effect of mood on retrieval is less obvious (Bower, 1987).

Consistent with this latter observation, the only study to date to examine the effects of state anxiety manipulations on memory for threat found no relationship (Foa, McNally, & Murdock, 1989). These researchers selected speech-anxious subjects, asked them to rate the personal applicability of a number of adjectives, and then gave them an unexpected recall task. In a 2 × 2 design, subjects were either anxious or not anxious at either adjective rating or recall. There was no effect of state anxiety, either during learning or recall, on the proportion of anxiety words recalled.

Another study in which state anxiety levels were manipulated has implications for memory organization (Butler & Mathews, 1987). In this study, students high and low in trait anxiety were asked both 1 month and 1 day before an important exam to indicate the probability that various events would happen to them. The results indicated that as the exam approached there was an increase in the perceived likelihood of negative events, but only those related to the exam. As described above, such data imply that an increase in the availability of information related to specific threat accompanies increases in state anxiety.

Finally, evidence on the accessibility of information related to lack of control in high GA has not yet been obtained. Questionnaire studies have certainly indicated that anxious patients believe they have less control in general than do nonanxious controls or stress-disordered patients (Rapee, Craske, & Barlow, 1989). In addition, there exists considerable laboratory work with animals indicating that learned information about control can influence anxious responding (e.g., see Barlow, 1988). However, direct evidence on the representation of control information and its role in GA will have to await future research.

Working Memory

Baddeley and Hitch (1974) summarized a series of studies indicating the value of describing a unique memory system for the short-term storing and processing of information, which they termed "working memory." Although there is still controversy over the necessity of defining multiple, unique memory systems (Humphreys, Bain, & Pike, 1989), the widespread use of the concept of working memory and the intuitive relevance of this concept for GAD (see below) suggest that it is worth discussing separately.

The central and most defining aspect of GAD is the tendency to worry (Rapee, in press; see also Chapter 2, this volume). Borkovec (1985; Borkovec, Robinson, Pruzinsky, & De Pree, 1983) has described worry as being uncontrollable, laden with negative affect, verbal, and aimed at attempted problem solving. For example, in a recent study, Borkovec and Inz (1990) found that worrying was associated with a predominance of thought (verbal) activity rather than images. To this description of worry, I have added elsewhere (Rapee, in press) that it is also conscious and attention-demanding.

Examination of this description of worry indicates a close fit between many of the features of worry and the descriptive aspects of working memory (Baddeley, 1990; Baddeley & Hitch, 1974). Thus it can be tentatively suggested that when it occurs, worry largely utilizes the resources of working memory (Rapee, in press). In particular, the conscious, verbal, attention-demanding, and problem-solving aspects of worry point to working memory. Working memory has been hypothesized to consist of at least three subsystems: two "slave" subsystems (the phonological loop and visual–spatial sketchpad) and a "controlling" subsystem (the central executive) (Baddeley, 1990). The phonological loop and visual–spatial sketchpad are involved in the simple manipulation of speech-based and visual–spatial information, respectively; the central executive plays a supervisory role, being responsible for the allocation of attentional resources. The description of worry provided above, together with the recent evidence by Borkovec and Inz (1990) that worry involves more thought than visual activity, points specifically to the central executive and the phonological loop as the most likely mediating structures for worry (Rapee, in press).

Empirical investigation of the mediation of worry through working memory is presently nonexistent, but a few studies have investigated important related issues. Borkovec et al. (1983) found that following a 15-minute period of voluntary worrying, both self-reported worriers and nonworriers had difficulty focusing their attention on a neutral stimulus (their breathing). Thus, it appears that worry is certainly attention-demanding and difficult to "switch-off." In a later, similar study, speech-anxious subjects were asked to engage in either worrying, neutral behavior, or relaxation behavior immediately prior to imaginal exposure to a fearful situation (giving a speech) (Borkovec & Hu, 1990). Heart rate from baseline to scene presentation was found to increase in both the neutral and relaxation conditions, but showed no change in the worry condition (baseline heart rate was equivalent across groups). The authors suggested that worrying serves somehow to reduce emotional processing. However, the results in fact can be interpreted in much the same way as in the Borkovec et al. (1983) study: Worrying in these anxious subjects was so attention-demanding that they were unable to switch all attentional processes to the phobic scene.

In another study, Eysenck (1985) asked subjects high and low in trait anxiety to solve two letter transformation tasks, differing in complexity. High-anxiety subjects performed worse than low-anxiety subjects on the more complex task, a robust finding. More importantly, further investigation indicated that the poorer performance in high-anxiety subjects was a result of difficulties with verbal rehearsal and storage. Eysenck suggested that anxiety reduces performance through its effect on working memory, especially the central executive.

Self-Schemas

The final issue to discuss in relation to information processing in GA is the role of self-schemas. "Self-schemas" are structures that organize information related to the self. Self-schemas are thought to play a role in the maintenance of depression (Segal, 1988), and the question thus arises as to whether they may also play a mediating role in GA. If this is so, then it would suggest that anxious individuals allocate attention to and efficiently process information specifically related to threat to the self. Strong support for this hypothesis comes from the study by Butler and Mathews (1983), in which they examined subjective probabilities for various events reported by subjects with GA and nonanxious individuals. This study demonstrated that anxious subjects reported a higher probability for threatening events than did nonanxious controls, but only for threatening events happening to themselves. Anxious subjects did not perceive a greater likelihood than nonanxious subjects for threatening events happening to someone else. A similar effect, although not quite as strong, appeared to occur with state anxiety (Butler & Mathews, 1987). Specifically, immediately before an examination, anxious subjects perceived a higher probability for negative events related to the examination for themselves, but not for someone else taking the same examination.

Unfortunately, more objective studies of this phenomenon have not been adequately conducted. In an early study using students high and low in social anxiety, subjects listened to tape-recorded trait adjectives under four conditions varying the depth of processing (Smith, Ingram, & Brehm, 1983). The four levels of processing were as follows: structural (was the word read by a male or female voice?), semantic (was the word the same as another?), private self-referent (did the word describe the individual?), and public self-referent (would another person say that the word described the individual?). High-anxiety subjects recalled significantly greater number of words only in the public self-referent condition, providing some evidence for the importance of self-schema in anxious processing. Given that the subjects were socially anxious, the importance of a public self-referent condition ("what others think of me") is not especially surprising. Perhaps generally anxious subjects would show more of a private self-referent effect.

However, the only studies conducted have failed to demonstrate a self-referent bias in anxiety on tests of memory (Mogg et al., 1987; Mogg & Mathews, 1990). Of course, as discussed earlier, the effects of anxiety on long-term memory per se have not been conclusive. In the earlier study (Mogg et al., 1987), GAD patients and controls judged threat-related and non-threat-related words and were then presented with unexpected recall and recognition tasks. The initial word judgments were of two types: Subjects had to decide whether the word described themselves or described a famous television personality. If self-schema are used to aid recall of threat-related words, then improved retrieval of threat-related words should only have been found in the self-referent condition for anxious patients. Overall, the results indicated a greater number of words remembered by both groups in the self-judgment condition. However, there was no significant interaction among judgment condition, word type, and diagnostic group.

In the second study (Mogg & Mathews, 1990), GAD patients and nonanxious controls were asked to rate the degree to which anxiety-related and non-anxiety-related adjectives described either themselves or the average person. They were warned that they would be tested on recall, which may have increased the influence of IQ, memory, or motivation. The words were also *anxiety*-related adjectives (such as "nervous") rather than *threat*-related words. Anxious subjects did not recall more anxiety-related adjectives in the self-referent than in the other condition.

Thus, these data appear to suggest that self-schemas are not specifically influential in the processing of threat information in anxiety, at least as far as recall and recognition are concerned. However, given the confusing results found with memory studies of anxious patients in general, this may not be surprising. Furthermore, self-schemas may still prove to be important in anxiety, but they may be found to influence only attention and initial processing, not retrieval.

CONCLUSIONS

GAD as a problem in its own right has not been recognized until relatively recently. As a result, research into the nature, etiology, and maintenance of GAD has not been extensive. Much of the work described above has come from one or two centers, and most of the conclusions have been derived from work on GA (chronic anxiety, trait anxiety). Although GA and GAD overlap to a considerable extent, they are not necessarily identical, and this must be kept in mind when evaluating the research on GA. Some interesting suggestions, especially in respect to the maintenance of GAD, are beginning to emerge, but at the current state of investigation these suggestions must remain tentative.

In sum, the bulk of the evidence appears to suggest that high GA is characterized by information processing that differs from that of nonanxious individuals. Further research may well indicate that this information processing is more realistic than that of normals in certain circumstances, much as has been shown with depression. Nevertheless, it differs from "normal" processing in a number of ways.

Two basic constructs are likely to be important in the maintenance of high GA and thus probably in GAD: biased perceptions of threat, and general perceptions of uncontrollability. Chronically anxious individuals appear to focus a greater number of attentional resources on potential threat than do nonanxious individuals. In addition, they seem to have more elaborated or active schemas for such information, as indicated by such features as threatening interpretations of ambiguous stimuli and better memory for threat-related information (at least at an implicit level). There is currently less evidence of this nature for the importance of uncontrollability-related information. However, at least one study has indicated the importance of uncontrollability in the environment for the development of fearful behavior in monkeys, and questionnaire studies have demonstrated that GAD subjects score lower on measures of perceived controllability than do nonanxious controls. Clearly, this latter factor requires considerable investigation to determine its ultimate role in the maintenance of GAD.

Given the limited empirical investigations of psychological factors involved in GA and GAD, the main aim of the present chapter has been to provide a framework in which to conceptualize the current evidence and to indicate important directions for future research. The information-processing model used here appears promising as a scheme into which to place emerging pieces of the puzzle. Let us hope that the next few years will see an increased interest in research into this fundamental aspect of human emotion.

REFERENCES

American Psychiatric Assocation. (1980). *Diagnostic and statistical manual of mental disorders* (3rd ed.). Washington, DC: Author.

American Psychiatric Assocation. (1987). *Diagnostic and statistical manual of mental disorders* (3rd ed., rev.). Washington, DC: Author.

Baddeley, A. D. (1990). *Human memory: Theory and practice*. London: Allyn & Bacon.

Baddeley, A. D., & Hitch, G. (1974). Working memory. In G. H. Bower (Ed.), *The psychology of learning and motivation: Advances in research and theory*. New York: Academic Press.

Barlow, D. H. (1988). *Anxiety and its disorders: The nature and treatment of anxiety and panic*. New York: Guilford Press.

Barlow, D. H., Blanchard, E. B., Vermilyea, J. A., Vermilyea, B. B., & Di Nardo, P. A. (1986). Generalized anxiety and generalized anxiety disorder: Description and reconceptualization. *American Journal of Psychiatry, 143*, 40–44.

Beck, A. T., Emery, G., & Greenberg, R. (1985). *Anxiety disorders and phobias: A cognitive perspective*. New York: Basic Books.

Beck, A. T., Laude, R., & Bohnert, M. (1974). Ideational components of anxiety neurosis. *Archives of General Psychiatry, 31*, 319–325.

Borkovec, T. D. (1985). Worry: A potentially valuable concept. *Behaviour Research and Therapy, 23*, 481–482.

Borkovec, T. D., & Hu, S. (1990). The effect of worry on cardiovascular response to phobic imagery. *Behaviour Research and Therapy, 28,* 69–73.

Borkovec, T. D., & Inz, J. (1990). The nature of worry in generalized anxiety disorder: A predominance of thought activity. *Behaviour Research and Therapy, 28,* 153–158.

Borkovec, T. D., Robinson, E., Pruzinsky, T., & DePree, J. A. (1983). Preliminary exploration of worry: Some characteristics and processes. *Behaviour Research and Therapy, 21,* 9–16.

Bower, G. H. (1981). Mood and memory. *American Psychologist, 36,* 129–148.

Bower, G. H. (1987). Commentary on mood and memory. *Behaviour Research and Therapy, 25,* 443–445.

Brewer, W. F., & Nakamura, G. V. (1984). The nature and functions of schemas. In R. S. Wyer & T. K. Srull (Eds.), *Handbook of social cognition* (Vol. 1). Hillsdale, NJ: Erlbaum.

Broadbent, D., & Broadbent, M. (1988). Anxiety and attentional bias: State and trait. *Cognition and Emotion, 2,* 165–183.

Butler, G., & Mathews, A. (1983). Cognitive processes in anxiety. *Advances in Behaviour Research and Therapy, 5,* 51–62.

Butler, G., & Mathews, A. (1987). Anticipatory anxiety and risk perception. *Cognitive Therapy and Research, 11,* 551–565.

Easterbrook, J. A. (1959). The effect of emotion on cue utilization and the organization of behavior. *Psychological Review, 66,* 183–201.

Eysenck, M. W. (1985). Anxiety and cognitive task performance. *Personality and Individual Differences, 6,* 579–586.

Eysenck, M. W., & Mathews, A. (1987). Trait anxiety and cognition. In H. J. Eysenck & I. Martin (Eds.), *Theoretical foundations of behavior therapy.* New York: Plenum.

Foa, E. B., McNally, R., & Murdock, T. B. (1989). Anxious mood and memory. *Behaviour Research and Therapy, 27,* 141–147.

Fridlund, A. J., Hatfield, M. E., Cottam, G. L., & Fowler, S. C. (1986). Anxiety and striate muscle activation: Evidence from electromyographic pattern analysis. *Journal of Abnormal Psychology, 95,* 228–236.

Hibbert, G. A. (1984). Ideational components of anxiety: Their origin and content. *British Journal of Psychiatry, 144,* 618–624.

Hoehn-Saric, R. (1981). Characteristics of chronic anxiety patients. In D. F. Klein & J. Rabkin (Eds.), *Anxiety: New research and changing concepts.* New York: Raven Press.

Hope, D. A., Rapee, R. M., Heimberg, R. G., & Dombeck, M. J. (1990). Representations of the self in social phobia: Vulnerability to social threat. *Cognitive Therapy and Research, 14,* 177–189.

Humphries, M. S., Bain, J. D., & Pike, R. (1989). Different ways to cue a coherent memory system: A theory for episodic, semantic, and procedural tasks. *Psychological Review, 96,* 208–233.

Kahneman, D. (1973). *Attention and effort.* Englewood Cliffs, NJ: Prentice-Hall.

Lader, M. (1972). The nature of anxiety. *British Journal of Psychiatry, 121,* 481–491.

Lazarus, R. S. (1966). *Psychological stress and the coping process*. New York: McGraw-Hill.

MacLeod, C., & Mathews, A. (1988). Anxiety and the allocation of attention to threat. *Quarterly Journal of Experimental Psychology, 40A*, 653–670.

MacLeod, C., Mathews, A., & Tata, P. (1986). Attentional bias in emotional disorders. *Journal of Abnormal Psychology, 95*, 15–20.

Marks, I. M., & Lader, M. (1973). Anxiety states (anxiety neurosis): A review. *Journal of Nervous and Mental Disease, 156*, 3–16.

Martin, M., Williams, R., & Clark, D. M. (1988). *Does anxiety lead to selective processing of theat-related information?* Paper presented at the World Congress of Behaviour Therapy, Edinburgh.

Mathew, R. J., Ho, B. T., Kralik, P., Taylor, D. L., & Claghorn, J. L. (1981). Catecholamines and monoamine oxidase activity in anxiety. *Acta Psychiatrica Scandinavica, 63*, 245–252.

Mathews, A., & MacLeod, C. (1985). Selective processing of threat cues in anxiety states. *Behaviour Research and Therapy, 23*, 563–569.

Mathews, A., & MacLeod, C. (1986). Discrimination of threat cues without awareness in anxiety states. *Journal of Abnormal Psychology, 95*, 131–138.

Mathews, A., & MacLeod, C. (1987). An information-processing approach to anxiety. *Journal of Cognitive Psychotherapy, 1*, 24–30.

Mathews, A., Mogg, K., May, J., & Eysenck, M. W. (1989). Implicit and explicit memory biases in anxiety. *Journal of Abnormal Psychology, 98*, 236–240.

Mathews, A., Richards, A., & Eysenck, M. (1989). Interpretation of homophones related to threat in anxiety states. *Journal of Abnormal Psychology, 98*, 31–34.

Mineka, S., Gunnar, M., & Champoux, M. (1986). Control and early socioemotional development: Infant rhesus monkeys reared in controllable and uncontrollable environments. *Child Developments, 57*, 1241–1256.

Mogg, K., & Mathews, A. (1990). Is there a self-referent mood-congruent recall bias in anxiety? *Behaviour Research and Therapy, 28*, 91–92.

Mogg, K., & Mathews, A., & Weinman, J. (1987). Memory bias in clinical anxiety. *Journal of Abnormal Psychology, 96*, 94–98.

Rapee, R. (1985). Distinctions between panic disorder and generalised anxiety disorder: Clinical presentation. *Australian and New Zealand Journal of Psychiatry, 19*, 227–232.

Rapee, R. M. (in press). Generalized anxiety disorder: A review of clinical features and theoretical concepts. *Clinical Psychology Review*.

Rapee, R. M., Craske, M. G., & Barlow, D. H. (1989). *A questionnaire to assess perceived control over emotions*. Paper presented at the 23rd Annual Meeting of the Association for Advancement of Behavior Therapy, Washington, DC.

Raskin, M., Peeke, H. V. S., Dickman, W., & Pinsker, H. (1982). Panic and generalized anxiety disorders. *Archives of General Psychiatry, 39*, 687–689.

Segal, Z. V. (1988). Appraisal of the self-schema construct in cognitive models of depression. *Psychological Bulletin, 103*, 147–162.

Smith, T. W., Ingram, R. E., & Brehm, S. S. (1983). Social anxiety, anxious self-preoccupation, and recall of self-relevant information. *Journal of Personality* and Social Psychology, 44, 1276–1283.

Spielberger, C. D. (1972). Anxiety as an emotional state. In C. D. Spielberger (Ed.), Anxiety: Current trends in theory and research. New York: Academic Press.

Stroop, J. R. (1935). Studies of interference in serial verbal reactions. Journal of Experimental Psychology, 18, 643–662.

Taylor, J. A. (1951). The relationship of anxiety to the conditioned eyelid response. Journal of Experimental Psychology, 41, 81–92.

Torgersen, S. (1986). Childhood and family characteristics in panic and generalized anxiety disorders. American Journal of Psychiatry, 143, 630–632.

Tversky, A., & Kahneman, D. (1974). Judgement under uncertainty: Heuristics and biases in judgements reveal some heuristics of thinking under uncertainty. Science, 185, 1124–1131.

Yerkes, R. M., & Dodson, J. D. (1908). The relation of strength of stimulus to rapidity of habit-formation. Journal of Comparative Neurology and Psychology, 18, 459–482.

Wolpe, J. (1958). Psychotherapy by reciprocal inhibition. Stanford, CA: Stanford University Press.

5

The Diagnosis of Generalized Anxiety Disorder: Development, Current Status, and Future Directions

DAVID H. BARLOW
PETER A. DI NARDO
University at Albany, State University of New York

Anxiety has always been part of the human condition. And yet we are only now beginning to describe anxiety and its disorders in a meaningful and useful manner. Formal attempts to classify psychopathology, including anxiety disorders, did not begin to appear until close to 1950. The term "anxiety" did not appear in the *International Classification of Diseases* (ICD) until the seventh revision, published in 1955. At that time the listing was "anxiety reaction without mention of somatic symptoms" under the general heading of "psychoneurotic disorders" (Jablensky, 1985).

Early attempts to classify anxiety disorders were deeply influenced by prevailing theoretical conceptions. When describing what we would now call "generalized anxiety," the prevailing conception was very clearly subsumed within the term "neurosis." Automatically, this shifted the focus from the observable features of anxiety disorders to hypothetical underlying unconscious conflicts maintaining the anxiety. Several developments led to deletion of the term "neurosis" with the publication of the *Diagnostic and Statistical Manual of Mental Disorders*, third edition (DSM-III; American Psychiatric Association, 1980). First, new theories regarding etiology and maintaining factors for anxiety disorders were suggested. Some of these were biological; others were based on psychological and social learning concepts that departed from specific theoretical conceptions underlying the term "neurosis." Second, many pointed out that the term "neurosis" did not facilitate research and classification, mostly because the term was too general and could not be defined reliably. This generality also contributed to difficulties with the usefulness or validity of the concept.

Of course, the term "neurosis" subsumed many disorders not currently included among the anxiety disorders in DSM-III or DSM-III-R (American Psychiatric Association, 1987). Beginning with DSM-III, only those neurotic disorders in which anxiety is experienced directly were grouped together as anxiety disorders. Remaining DSM-II neurotic disorders were distributed among other classes, such as somatoform disorders, dissociative disorders, and affective disorders.

Therefore, the disorder now referred to as "generalized anxiety disorder" (GAD) has undergone enormous change over the past several decades. This has caused substantial confusion among professionals and scientists. We have proceeded from DSM-II, where what is now GAD was subsumed under a single broad heading of "anxiety neurosis," to a very different definition today. Anxiety neurosis in DSM-II became "anxiety states (or anxiety neurosis)" in DSM-III and was subdivided into the newly defined panic disorder as well as GAD (along with obsessive compulsive disorder [OCD] and post-traumatic stress disorder). In DSM-III-R, the parenthetical "anxiety neurosis" was dropped altogether, and panic disorder was further subdivided into panic disorder either with or without agoraphobia. The DSM-II diagnosis "depressive neurosis" joined the affective or mood disorders in DSM-III and ultimately became dysthymia.

This process has clearly favored those nosologists who can be characterized as "splitters" rather than "lumpers." Splitters tend to subdivide categories into ever smaller units, achieving greater reliability, but at the expense (perhaps) of the usefulness of the system of classification. Nosological progress is a continual battle between the splitters and the lumpers. Models and evidence presented in previous chapters of this volume suggest that we may wish to reexamine what is common about anxiety and depression (anxiety neurosis and depressive neurosis), since these commonalities may ultimately provide a more useful basis for classification. The remainder of this chapter deals first with the development of the DSM-III-R classification of GAD. Following this, revisions to GAD criteria currently under consideration by the DSM-IV Subgroup on GAD and Mixed Anxiety–Depression are reviewed.

DSM-III GENERALIZED ANXIETY DISORDER

It is now widely agreed that the DSM-III category of GAD created enormous confusion. This was due primarily to its status as a residual category. That is, patients could not be diagnosed as having GAD unless they did not meet the criteria for any other anxiety or affective disorder. Diagnosis by exclusion, of course, is certain to produce fuzzy discriminations and difficult decisions. Such was the case with DSM-III GAD. Kappa coefficients reflecting the ability of two independent interviewers to agree on the presence or absence of GAD were characteristically low, compared to those for other anxiety disorders (Barlow, 1987, 1988). In our initial study, utilizing very conservative criteria, the kappa coefficient for 12 consecutive GAD patients out of a series of 125 consecutive admissions to our clinic diagnosed with anxiety disorders was .571 (Barlow, 1987). When we examined reasons for disagreement between these two independent interviewers, a number of possibilities emerged. But one cause for disagreement unique to GAD was an inability to determine whether GAD was severe enough to be classified as a disorder. In other words, a number of people would present with sufficient symptoms of anxiety lasting 1 month or more (the DSM-III criterion), but the interviewers would disagree as to whether the anxiety was severe enough to warrant labeling it a disorder (DiNardo, O'Brien, Barlow, Waddell, & Blanchard, 1983).

Conceptualizing GAD as a residual disorder implies that the symptoms of generalized anxiety are in fact present in the remaining anxiety disorders, but that these disorders have something "in addition" to generalized anxiety, such as panic attacks or intrusive thoughts. To test this, we examined for DSM-III GAD symptoms across a variety of anxiety disorders as well as major depression (Barlow, Blanchard, Vermilyea, Vermilyea, & Di Nardo, 1986). Some of these results are presented in Table 5.1, which contains the mean severity ratings for the four DSM-III GAD symptom clusters rated within each anxiety disorder category. Although patients with GAD had arithmetically higher severity ratings for two of the four symptom clusters (muscle tension and autonomic hyperactivity), in no instance did the difference between ratings across groups reach statistical significance.

Thus, it seems clear that almost all of these patients with anxiety disorders presented with the four basic features defining GAD in DSM-III. The one exception was the category of simple phobia, where only 40% met criteria for GAD. Even this proportion may be artifactually high for simple phobia, since very few patients come to our Phobia and Anxiety Disorders Clinic with simple phobia as their only problem. Most often, additional anxiety disorder or affective disorder diagnoses are assigned, even though simple phobia is the principal (most severe) diagnosis. It may be that in the case of simple phobia without additional problems, an even lower percentage of patients would meet the criteria for GAD. But very few of these people come in for treatment.

Not only did a relatively high proportion of each diagnostic category meet the criteria for GAD, but, as noted above, we were not able to

TABLE 5.1. Severity of Generalized Anxiety Disorder Symptoms for Each Primary Diagnosis of 99 Anxious Patients

	Severity of generalized anxiety disorder symptom clusters[a]							
	Muscle tension[b]		Autonomic hyperactivity[c]		Vigilance and scanning[d]		Apprehensive expectation[e]	
Primary diagnosis	Mean	SD	Mean	SD	Mean	SD	Mean	SD
Agoraphobia with panic ($n = 39$)[f]	1.46	0.908	1.95	0.804	1.81	0.775	2.22	0.785
Social phobia ($n = 17$)	1.53	1.138	1.62	0.993	1.85	0.897	2.12	0.839
Simple phobia ($n = 6$)	1.08	1.357	1.00	0.949	1.25	1.084	1.58	1.357
Panic disorder ($n = 17$)	1.56	0.796	2.04	0.705	1.78	0.825	2.25	0.925
Generalized anxiety disorder ($n = 11$)	2.18	0.902	2.18	0.513	1.81	0.751	1.77	0.876
Obsessive compulsive disorder ($n = 4$)	1.38	0.479	2.13	0.629	2.50	0.577	2.63	0.479
Major depressive episode ($n = 5$)	2.10	1.245	1.70	1.204	2.40	0.894	2.40	0.822

Note. From Barlow, D. H., Blanchard, E. B., Vermilyea, J. A., Vermilyea, B. B., & Di Nardo, P. A. (1986). Generalized anxiety and generalized anxiety disorder: Description and reconceptualization. *American Journal of Psychiatry, 143,* 40–44. Copyright 1986 by the American Psychiatric Association. Reprinted by permission.

[a] $0 =$ none, $1 =$ mild, $2 =$ moderate, $3 =$ severe, $4 =$ very severe.

[b] $F = 1.34$, $df = 6, 90$, n.s.

[c] $F = 1.92$, $df = 6, 91$, n.s.

[d] $F = 1.36$, $df = 6, 92$, n.s.

[e] $F = 1.13$, $df = 6, 92$, n.s.

[f] For muscle tension, $n = 37$; for autonomic hyperactivity, $n = 38$.

discriminate reliably among the various anxiety disorders on the basis of severity ratings for GAD symptom clusters. Thus, DSM-III GAD met the requirement of a "residual" category, in that symptoms of GAD were found in all of the remaining anxiety disorder categories. On the basis of these data, there seemed little reason to note the existence of GAD symptoms, with the possible exception of cases where simple phobia was the principal diagnosis.

THE DEVELOPMENT OF DSM-III-R GAD

Nevertheless, clinical experience suggested that a number of patients successfully treated at our clinic for one or another of the anxiety disorders (e.g., agoraphobia) continued to experience severe discomfort as a result of more generalized anxiety, even after treatment had concluded. Others did not. It seemed that the former individuals were suffering from generalized anxiety that was independent of their presenting disorder. On the basis of these observations it seemed that GAD could be conceptualized as a separate anxiety disorder category, diagnosable in addition to other anxiety disorders. We accomplished this by differentiating between the anticipatory anxiety that is almost always part of a panic or phobic disorder, and generalized anxiety. More precisely, we found that it was important to ascertain the cognitive focus of patients' anxiety—that is, what they were worrying about. Was their worry focused on the next panic attack or phobic encounter (anticipatory anxiety), or was it focused on other areas?

Part of the evidence supporting this strategy of ascertaining cognitive focus came from a study (Barlow, Di Nardo, Vermilyea, Vermilyea, & Blanchard, 1986) in which patients were assigned all of the DSM-III anxiety and affective disorder diagnoses for which they qualified. In other words, the diagnostic exclusionary rules that were part of DSM-III procedures were dropped. This practice allows the establishment of patterns of comorbidity. An updated description of comorbidity among the anxiety disorders is presented in Chapter 6. What was surprising to us in the Barlow, Di Nardo, et al. (1986) study, in light of the prevalence of GAD symptom clusters noted above, was how few additional diagnoses of GAD were assigned when the principal diagnosis was another anxiety disorder, such as social phobia or panic disorder.

From the data presented in Table 5.1, one would assume that GAD would be a very common additional diagnosis. The reason it was not had to do with the way diagnoses were made in that study. In making a decision as to whether an additional diagnosis of GAD was warranted, clinicians determined whether symptoms of GAD were an associated feature or an integral part of the principal diagnosis, or whether they represented a coexisting independent problem. In order to make this determination with GAD symptoms, clinicians had to determine the focus of apprehensive expectation—one of the four symptom clusters of GAD. In other words, what were the patients worrying about? If they were worrying about the next panic attack, or perhaps their next encounter with a socially phobic situation (depending on their principal diagnosis), this would be anticipatory anxiety and was judged as such by our clinicians. Anticipatory anxiety is, of course, an integral part or associated feature of a principal diagnosis of phobia or panic disorder. However, if the focus of apprehensive expectation was on multiple life circumstances (many of which were unrelated to the principal diagnosis), and the patients also presented with the other three symptom clusters (muscle tension, autonomic hyperactivity, and vigilance or scanning), an additional diagnosis of GAD was assigned. In this case, GAD would be a coexisting independent problem. This required a determination of the functional relationship among anxiety features. This practice, along with fully establishing patterns of comorbidity, has been incorporated into the revisions of DSM-III.

In devising a new definition of GAD based on the considerations described above, we thought it best to work with a conservative definition at first. For that reason, we required identification of two general areas or life situations that were serving as the focus of chronic apprehensive expectation. We recognized that future research might demonstrate that only one "sphere of worry" was necessary and sufficient to discriminate the syndrome of GAD (see below). But requiring identification of two spheres of worry would separate the problem more clearly from other anxiety disorders and ensure that this anxiety is truly "generalized."

Thus, we came to the conclusion that the cardinal feature of GAD was specified in DSM-III as apprehensive expectation. Distinguishing a syndrome of GAD from the anticipatory anxiety often found in other anxiety disorders depends on determining the focus of apprehensive expectation or worry. When this is done, a group of patients emerge who can be characterized as "chronic worriers," with sufficient severity ratings and accompanying somatic symptoms to meet criteria for GAD. Conceptualizing GAD in this way removes it as a residual category and bases classification on a cardinal symptom not necessarily present in other anxiety disorders. This strategy is consistent with our experience (and that of other clinicians) that chronic pathological and diffuse "worrying" does not necessarily covary with symptoms of other anxiety disorders during treatment, such as panic or intrusive thoughts. These conceptualizations form the basis for the DSM-III-R category of GAD.

Clinicians working with DSM-III definitions of GAD also reported difficulty in setting the duration criterion at 1 month. Many pointed out, correctly, that experience with any number of negative life events may produce temporary adjustment reactions lasting a month or more and consisting of the DSM-III symptom clusters. Although these reactions result in only temporary emotional distress, they technically qualify as DSM-III GAD if the duration is 1 month or more. Breslau and Davis (1985) examined the utility of extending the duration criterion to 6 months. Using both 1-month and 6-month duration criteria, they found that the latter cut prevalence rates dramatically in 357 women surveyed from the general population. Specifically, prevalence rates were reduced from a (very high) estimate of 11.5% to 2.4%. Extending the duration to 6 months also yielded a group of patients who reported a greater number of symptoms, as well as more severe symptoms. Thus, extending the duration to 6 months seemed to approximate more closely the popular clinical conception of GAD as *excess* anxiety experienced *chronically*. (This is consistent with data on duration of GAD in patients who seek help at specialty clinics, where chronicity of several years or more is the rule.) This extension also had the virtue of allowing adjustment reactions to last up to 6 months without overlapping with GAD. For all these reasons, the 6-month criterion was adopted for DSM-III-R. DSM-III and DSM-III-R criteria for GAD are presented in Table 5.2.

RECENT RESEARCH ON THE DSM-III-R GAD DEFINITION

In this section of the chapter, we examine the diagnostic reliability of DSM-III-R GAD, as well as the reliability of the specific symptom criteria that constitute the diagnosis.

As noted above, DSM-III-R includes several changes in the criteria for GAD that may have a significant impact on the reliability of the diagnosis. To review, the defining feature of GAD is now excessive or unrealistic worry in two spheres—a change that reflects a shift in emphasis from the somatic symptoms to the cognitive component of the disorder. The somatic symptom criteria have been retained in modified form, with a requirement of 6 of 18 symptoms from three areas: motor tension; autonomic hyperactivity; and vigilance and scanning. Apprehensive expectation has been eliminated because it is subsumed under the worry criterion.

As also described above, the hierarchical assumptions have been modified, and many automatic exclusions have been eliminated, increasing the number of instances of multiple diagnoses. GAD can be assigned as an additional diagnosis in the presence of another Axis I disorder, provided that the focus of worry is on two areas other than the Axis I disorder. In cases of mood or psychotic disorders, GAD is still automatically excluded

TABLE 5.2. DSM-III and DSM-III-R Diagnostic Criteria for GAD

DSM-III[a]	DSM-III-R[b]
A. Generalized, persistent anxiety is manifested by symptoms from three of the following four categories: (1) *motor tension*: shakiness, jitteriness, jumpiness, trembling, tension, muscle aches, fatigability, inability to relax, eyelid twitch, furrowed brow, strained face, fidgeting, restlessness, easy startle (2) *autonomic hyperactivity*: sweating, heart pounding or racing, cold clammy hands, dry mouth, dizziness, light-headedness, paresthesias (tingling in hands or feet), upset stomach, hot or cold spells, frequent urination, diarrhea, discomfort in the pit of the stomach, lump in the throat, flushing, pallor, high resting pulse and respiration rate (3) *apprehensive expectation*: anxiety, worry, fear, rumination, and anticipation of misfortune to self or others (4) *vigilance and scanning*: hyperattentiveness resulting in distractibility, difficulty in concentrating, insomnia, feeling "on edge," irritability, impatience	A. Unrealistic or excessive anxiety and worry (apprehensive expectation) about two or more life circumstances, e.g., worry about possible misfortune to one's child (who is in no danger) and worry about finances (for no good reason), for a period of six months or longer, during which the person has been bothered more days than not by these concerns. In children and adolescents, this may take the form of anxiety and worry about academic, athletic, and social performance.
B. The anxious mood has been continuous for at least one month.	B. If another Axis I disorder is present, the focus of the anxiety and worry in A is unrelated to it, e.g., the anxiety or worry is not about having a panic attack (as in Panic Disorder), being embarrassed in public (as in Social Phobia), being contaminated (as in Obsessive Compulsive Disorder), or gaining weight (as in Anorexia Nervosa).
C. Not due to another mental disorder, such as a Depressive Disorder or Schizophrenia.	C. The disturbance does not occur only during the course of a Mood Disorder or a psychotic disorder.

(cont.)

TABLE 5.2. (*Continued*)

DSM-III[a]	DSM-III-R[b]
D. At least 18 years of age.	D. At least 6 of the following 18 symptoms are often present when anxious (do not include symptoms present only during panic attacks):

Motor tension
- (1) trembling, twitching, or feeling shaky
- (2) muscle tension, aches, or soreness
- (3) restlessness
- (4) easy fatigability

Autonomic hyperactivity
- (5) shortness of breath or smothering sensations
- (6) palpitations or accelerated heart rate (tachycardia)
- (7) sweating, or cold clammy hands
- (8) dry mouth
- (9) dizziness or lightheadedness
- (10) nausea, diarrhea, or other abdominal distress
- (11) flushes (hot flashes) or chills
- (12) frequent urination
- (13) trouble swallowing or "lump in throat"

Vigilance and scanning
- (14) feeling keyed up or on edge
- (15) exaggerated startle response
- (16) difficulty concentrating or "mind going blank" because of anxiety
- (17) trouble falling or staying asleep
- (18) irritability

E. It cannot be established that an organic factor initiated and maintained the disturbance, e.g., hyperthyroidism, Caffeine Intoxication.

[a] Criteria from American Psychiatric Association. (1980). *Diagnostic and statistical manual of mental disorders* (3rd ed., p. 233). Washington, DC: Author. Copyright 1980 by the American Psychiatric Association. Reprinted by permission.
[b] Criteria from American Psychiatric Association. (1987). *Diagnostic and statistical manual of mental disorders* (3rd ed., rev., pp. 252–253). Washington, DC: Author. Copyright 1987 by the American Psychiatric Association. Reprinted by permission.

if the worry occurs only during the course of the mood or psychotic disorder.

The changes in the criteria are extensive, and can be expected to have significant impact on the frequency with which GAD is assigned, as well as the reliability of the diagnosis. For purposes of this chapter, research on the DSM-III definition of GAD is not relevant to questions of the reliability of the DSM-III-R category, other than as a comparison. However, since the final draft of DSM-III-R has only been available since early 1987, little research has appeared on the diagnostic reliability of DSM-III-R categories. This section focuses on the available research on the DSM-III-R revision of GAD, as well as on reports to the DSM-IV Subgroup on GAD and Mixed Anxiety–Depression, and on preliminary analyses of a data base relevant to GAD at our Center for Stress and Anxiety Disorders (CSAD) in Albany.

The Albany Data Base

Among our programs and clinics at the CSAD is an outpatient clinic specializing in the diagnosis and treatment of anxiety disorders (Phobia and Anxiety Disorders Clinic). As part of a National Institute of Mental Health project on the classification of anxiety disorders, a reliability study of the DSM-III-R anxiety disorder categories is currently in progress. As of this writing, 164 patients presented at the clinic and were diagnosed by two clinicians, who conducted independent interviews using the Anxiety Disorders Interview Schedule—Revised (ADIS-R; Di Nardo & Barlow, 1988). The ADIS-R is a structured interview protocol intended for differential diagnosis of DSM-III-R anxiety and mood disorders, with screening sections for other Axis I disorders. Elsewhere (Di Nardo, O'Brien, Barlow, Waddell, & Blanchard, 1983), we describe an earlier version of the interview and the reliability of DSM-III diagnoses derived from it (see also Barlow, 1987, 1988). After conducting separate interviews using the ADIS-R, the clinicians independently assigned principal diagnoses and any additional diagnoses, according to the DSM-III-R criteria. Kappa was calculated using the formula presented in Fleiss, Nee, and Landis (1979). For purposes of these calculations, agreement was defined as a match on the two interviewers' principal diagnoses. This is a very conservative definition, because both interviewers might identify GAD in a patient, but if one interviewer judged a coexisting disorder (e.g., major depressive episode [MDE]) as the more severe or "principal diagnosis," it would be scored a disagreement. Thus Interviewer 1 might have GAD as principal and MDE as additional, while Interviewer 2 would have MDE as principal and GAD as additional. This would be a disagreement despite the fact that both interviewers made both diagnoses. With this information in mind, we can review data collected at the CSAD and elsewhere on DSM-III-R GAD definitions.

Reliability of the GAD Diagnosis

Findings of the New York City and Albany Groups

Mannuzza et al. (1989) reported a study on the reliability of the DSM-III-R anxiety disorders using the SADS-LA, a modification of the Lifetime version of the Schedule for Affective Disorders and Schizophrenia. The SADS-LA is intended to cover the DSM-III-R anxiety and mood disorders, and yields both current and lifetime diagnoses. Subjects for this study were 104 individuals recruited from a pool of current and former anxiety disorder patients, most of whom were enrolled in research programs at the New York State Psychiatric Institute (NYSPI) Anxiety Disorders Clinic. Initially, 134 subjects agreed to participate, but 30 were eliminated because of (1) ongoing treatment at the NYSPI Depression Clinic, (2) being related to Anxiety Disorders Clinic patients, or (3) more than 60 days having elapsed between interviews. Each subject was interviewed on two separate occasions; one interview was conducted by an "expert" rater, who was not blind to the clinic diagnosis, and the other by a "field" rater. Expert raters were from the anxiety clinic staff, who demonstrated reliability on at least 13 SADS-LA interviews. Field raters were doctoral-level psychologists and social workers who had completed a training program in the SADS-LA. Diagnoses were assigned according to the *somatic* criteria for GAD in the October 5, 1985 working draft of DSM-III-R, and kappa was calculated separately for current (met criteria during the last 2 months) and lifetime (either a current or past episode) diagnoses. (Unfortunately, the SADS-LA did not include the "two spheres of worry" criterion that was included in the final DSM-III-R criteria for GAD.)

Additional kappas were calculated (e.g., to compare Research Diagnostic Criteria [RDC] and DSM diagnoses), but this review focuses on the current and lifetime anxiety disorder diagnoses. These kappas are presented in Table 5.3, together with the kappas from the CSAD data set. We have included kappas for all anxiety disorders, in order to provide a context in which to evaluate the reliability figures for GAD. Because of changes from the working draft to the final draft of DSM-III-R in the description of agoraphobic avoidance, the figures from the two sites for panic disorder and panic disorder with agoraphobia (PDA) cannot be directly compared, as is true of the figures for GAD.

For the CSAD data set, we present individual kappas for the three levels of avoidance in PDA. In addition, kappas were calculated for PDA when all levels of avoidance are combined, and for panic disorder plus

TABLE 5.3. Kappa Coefficients for DSM-III-R Anxiety Disorders

Diagnosis	Mannuzza et al. (1989) (n = 104)			CSAD (n = 164)		
	Lifetime	Current				
Panic disorder	.86 (63)	.79 (53)		.41 (20)		
Agoraphobia	.90 (45)	.81 (34)	PDA (mild)	.74 (58)	.79	.85
			PDA (moderate)	.78 (25)		
			PDA (severe)	.47 (6)		
Simple phobia	.29 (30)	.29 (30)		1.00 (5)		
Social phobia	.71 (52)	.68 (51)		.87 (32)		
OCD	.89 (17)	.91 (13)		.81 (13)		
GAD	.60 (15)	.27 (11)		.54 (22)		

Note. The Mannuzza et al. data are based on the October 5, 1985 working draft of DSM-III-R; the CSAD data are based on the final version. OCD, obsessive compulsive disorder; GAD, generalized anxiety disorder; PDA, panic disorder with agoraphobia. Numbers in parentheses refer to numbers of cases in which diagnosis was assigned by either or both raters.

PDA. The figures indicate that our interviewers had difficulty in applying some of the DSM-III-R descriptions of agoraphobic avoidance, but could readily agree on the presence of panic disorder. Mannuzza et al. (1989) obtained poor reliability for current GAD (.27), although the figure for lifetime GAD (.60) is in the "good" range. Mannuzza et al. suggest that the source of this difference was the inability of raters to agree on whether an episode was ongoing or remitted, though agreeing on the presence or absence of an episode at some time in the patient's life. In the CSAD sample, the kappa for GAD (.54) indicates fair agreement on current episodes. Although direct comparisons are difficult, use of the full DSM-III-R criteria may have contributed to improved reliability when compared to the Mannuzza et al. (1989) data on current episode. In addition, the reliance on DSM-III-R somatic symptoms may have been particularly problematic, in view of other uniformly poor reliabilities for these symptoms (see below). In both samples, the reliability of GAD is lower than that of the other anxiety disorders. The relatively low reliability of GAD compared to the other anxiety disorders was also reported in our earlier study (Di Nardo et al., 1983), using modified DSM-III criteria.

Sources of Disagreement

Mannuzza et al. (1989) used a consensus case conference to arrive at sources of diagnostic disagreement. For GAD, variance in subjects' reports of symptoms was identified as the source of disagreement in 57% of the cases. "Subject variance" refers to differences in the presence/absence or frequency and duration of specific symptoms reported to each interviewer. In the CSAD sample, agreement was defined only when there was a match on principal diagnosis, so disagreements can be characterized by examining the principal diagnosis assigned by the dissenting interviewer. Table 5.3 shows the distribution of principal diagnoses in the 13 cases of disagreement involving GAD. The table shows that in these cases there were a variety of alternate principal diagnoses, including the mood disorders. This could suggest that in some cases, interviewers found it difficult to distinguish GAD worry from worry that is an associated feature of other Axis I disorders. Two studies (Craske, Rapee, Jackel, & Barlow, 1989; Borkovec, et al., Chapter 2, this volume) have identified the content of GAD worry, and some of the spheres are similar to worries associated with other Axis I disorders: illness concerns, which are similar to those experienced by patients with somatoform disorders; interpersonal concerns, which may overlap with the evaluative fears experienced by patients with social phobia; and worries about the future, which may overlap with the pessimism associated with dysthymia.

The CSAD kappas presented in Table 5.3 are based on matches on principal dignosis. Table 5.4 also shows that in 7 of the 13 cases in which there was disagreement on principal diagnosis, the dissenting interviewer assigned GAD as an additional diagnosis. This indicates that both raters agreed that the patient met the criteria for a current GAD episode, independent of any other Axis I disorders; the only disagreement in these cases was whether GAD should be considered the principal diagnosis. If we recalculate kappa for GAD on the basis of the presence or absence of

TABLE 5.4. GAD Sources of Disagreement: Alternate Principal Diagnoses Assigned by Second Interviewer

Diagnosis	*n* of cases	GAD additional[a]
Panic disorder	1	1
PDA (mild)	1	1
Social phobia	3	3
Anxiety disorder not otherwise specified	1	0
MDE	2	0
Dysthymia	3	2
Somatoform	1	0
Adjustment disorder	1	0
Total	13	7

Note. MDE, major depressive episode.
[a]Number of cases in which GAD was assigned as an additional diagnosis.

the diagnosis, regardless of its status as principal or additional, the CSAD sample shows a kappa of .64 for GAD (GAD was assigned as principal or additional diagnosis by both raters in 57 cases, but by only one rater in 28 cases). This indicates that our raters were able to identify GAD as an independent diagnosis in cases in which another Axis I disorder was present.

One might speculate that the 28 cases involving GAD disagreement were more complex or diagnostically difficult. In order to examine this possibility, we compared the frequency and reliability of accompanying anxiety and mood disorder diagnoses in the 28 cases of GAD disagreement with those in the remaining 136 cases in which the interviewers agreed on the presence or absence of GAD. Table 5.5 shows that interviewers were about equally likely to assign anxiety disorder diagnoses in cases of GAD agreement and disagreement. The single exception is PDA (mild), which was assigned more frequently in disagreement cases (60.9%) than in agreement cases (35.3%). This suggests that the presence of PDA makes it more difficult to identify accompanying GAD, perhaps because the relatively greater severity of PDA compared to most other anxiety disorders (Barlow, 1988) makes it more difficult to determine whether an independent GAD exists. The answer must await a much closer and more detailed analysis.

The kappas for the additional diagnoses are quite interesting, although they must be interpreted with caution because of the small *n*. The kappas for the panic disorders are similar in the agreement and disagreement cases, but the kappas are lower for OCD and social phobia in the disagreement cases. These somewhat lower kappas require a closer look to determine whether interviewers were confusing the intrusive thoughts of OCD or

TABLE 5.5. Number (%) of Cases Receiving Additional Diagnoses in Cases of GAD Agreement and Disagreement

Diagnosis	Agreement (*n* = 136)	Disagreement (*n* = 28)
Panic disorder	22 (16.2)	5 (17.9)
PDA (mild)	48 (35.3)	17 (60.7)
PDA (moderate)	24 (17.6)	4 (14.3)
PDA (severe)	6 (4.6)	0 (0)
Simple phobia	56 (41.2)	13 (46.4)
Social phobia	75 (55.1)	16 (57.1)
OCD	21 (15.4)	3 (10.7)
MDE	33 (24.3)	5 (17.9)
Dysthymia	20 (14.7)	2 (7.1)

TABLE 5.6. Kappas for Additional Diagnoses in Cases of GAD Agreement and Disagreement

Diagnosis	Agreement ($n = 136$)	Disagreement ($n = 28$)
Panic disorder	.53	.58
PDA (mild)	.69	.64
PDA (moderate)	.73	.84
PDA (severe)	.48	—
Simple phobia	.50	.44
Social phobia	.63	.42
OCD	.65	.46
MDE	.58	.87
Dysthymia	.41	.65

evaluation concerns of social phobia with alternative spheres of worry that would indicate GAD. In view of the very high comorbidity between GAD and social phobia (see also Chapter 2), this could be an important source of confusion. We have already noted elsewhere (Craske et al., 1989) that emphasizing the worry component in DSM-III-R GAD may create a boundary problem with OCD.

Agreement on mood disorders was higher in cases of GAD disagreement. Taken together, the figures in Tables 5.5 and 5.6 concerning mood disorders show that interviewers were less likely to assign a mood disorder diagnosis in cases of GAD disagreement, but that when they did assign a mood disorder diagnosis, they were more likely to agree on it. It could be that in these cases with a clear, agreed-upon mood disorder, there was some worry or chronic anxiety that one interviewer subsumed under the mood disorder, while the other interviewer judged the worry to warrant a separate GAD diagnosis. This type of disagreement would only apply to some cases of GAD, because in general the presence of a mood disorder does not lower the reliability of GAD. For example, in the CSAD sample, there were 52 cases in which either or both raters assigned a diagnosis of MDE or dysthymia. In these cases, GAD was assigned by both raters as either principal or additional in 25 cases, but by only one rater in 7 cases, resulting in a kappa of .73. This indicates that our raters were able to discriminate GAD diagnoses reliably from depressive diagnoses.

In summary, then, the presence of a mood disorder does not lower reliability (in fact, it may sharpen it). But the presence of PDA seems to be associated with lower reliabilities for GAD. The presence of OCD or social phobia, on the other hand, is not associated specifically with lower kappas for GAD; however, when these diagnoses do accompany a GAD diagnosis where a disagreement occurred, the kappas for OCD and social phobias are also lower, suggesting a possible source of confusion. Firm answers will have to await more fine-grained analysis.

Reliability of GAD Symptom Ratings

In this section, we review studies that have reported reliability figures for symptom ratings constituting part of the DSM-III-R criteria for GAD, and we also report analyses of the CSAD data set. We consider ratings of physical symptoms of anxiety as described in criterion D, and ratings of spheres of excessive or unrealistic worry as described in criterion A.

Physical Symptoms

In a companion article to Mannuzza et al. (1989), Fyer et al. (1989) report on the reliability of "subdisorder" anxiety symptoms in the same sample used in the Mannuzza et al. article. This study focused on symptoms central to DSM-III-R anxiety disorders that were not sufficiently intense or frequent to meet disorder criteria. For the 18 physical symptoms of anxiety, separate kappas were calculated on ratings for the entire sample of patients and for a subgroup of patients who did not meet the criteria for a DSM-III-R GAD diagnosis. In the CSAD sample, the 18 symptoms were rated on a 5-point severity scale, and reliability was assessed by calculating Pearson r on the severity ratings of the two interviewers for each of the symptoms. Because the ADIS-R includes "skip out" questions, the ratings of physical symptoms were obtained only when the interviewer had judged criterion A (persistent, excessive worry) to be present or probably present. As a result, this sample includes patients who received a GAD diagnosis, as well as those whose symptoms did not meet the full GAD criteria; thus, our figures are more nearly comparable with the Fyer et al. (1989) figures for the total sample. Table 5.7 shows the Fyer et al. kappas (total sample) and the CSAD correlations for the 18 symptoms. For some symptoms the two studies used slightly different descriptors, and in these cases the ADIS-R descriptor appears in parentheses. Also, the symptom lists for the two interview protocols do not completely match. Each one contains items that do not appear in the other.

Despite differences in the manner in which the ratings were obtained and analyzed, there is striking consistency in their poor reliability. In the Fyer et al. sample, kappas ranged from .08 to .48, while correlations in the CSAD sample ranged from .05 to .63. Even worse, the symptoms showing the best reliability in one sample often showed poor reliability in the other sample. Fyer et al. attribute the poor reliability to variance in

TABLE 5.7. Reliability of GAD Criterion Symptoms

Symptom		Fyer et al. (1989)	CSAD
SADS-LA	ADIS-R	(kappa)	(Pearson r)
Jittery or jumpy	(Keyed up)	.34	.24
Shaky or trembling	Same	.30	.39
Muscles tense or achy	Same	.54	.19
Restlessness	Same	.40	.29
Easy fatiguability	Same	.26	.48
Sweating a lot	Same	.19	.38
Palpitations	Same	.34	.27
Dry mouth	Same	.16	.63
Dizzy or lightheaded	Same	.46	.28
Upset stomach/diarrhea	Same	.48	.48
Urinary frequency	Same	.46	.41
Lump in throat	Same	.44	.05
Flushed or pale	Same	.32	.33
Trouble concentrating	Same	.08	.22
Difficulty sleeping	Same	.27	.60
Irritability	Same	.36	.36
Eyelid twitching[a]	—	.41	—
Clammy hands[a]	—	.21	—
—	Startle easily[b]	—	.29
—	Short of breath[b]	—	.41

[a] Items appearing only in SADS-IA.
[b] Items appearing only in ADIS-R.

subjects' reports to the two raters. We have no systematic data on sources of disagreement on GAD symptoms, but our impression is that the variation in reports may be due to patients' difficulty in recalling experiences of specific symptoms over a 6-month period.

Excessive or Unrealistic Worry

Criterion A of DSM-III-R describes the essential feature of GAD as unrealistic and/or excessive anxiety or worry about two or more life circumstances. This criterion requires the clinician to identify the content of the worry (e.g., family, finances), and to determine whether the worry is excessive. Fyer et al. (1989) report a kappa of .42 for ratings of persistent anxiety of ⩾6 months, as defined in DSM-III criterion A. This definition is quite different from the DSM-III-R definition, and it is not clear whether Fyer et al. specifically included excessive/unrealistic worry in two spheres in their ratings of this criterion.

In order to examine the reliability of worry content, we (Craske et al., 1989) had 19 GAD patients and 26 normal controls fill out a worry questionnaire as soon as possible after they noticed themselves worrying. Two independent raters then categorized the worries into five spheres: (1) family/home and interpersonal relationships; (2) finances; (3) work/school; (4) illness/injury/health; and (5) miscellaneous (e.g., car transmission problems, breaking a plate, being late for an appointment). The raters agreed on categorization of 81.8% of the 44 worries reported by the GAD patients, and on 74.2% of the 62 worries reported by the controls. In addition, the worries reported by GAD patients on the questionnaire were compared with worries reported to an interviewer during the GAD section of the ADIS-R and rated by the interviewer as excessive/unrealistic. Two raters attained an agreement of 91.2% in categorizing the content of these worries into the five spheres noted above. This level of agreement is particularly striking in view of the different methods of obtaining the worry content.

In another study on the reliability of identification of worry content, Sanderson and Barlow (1990) used the ADIS-R to conduct independent interviews on 14 GAD patients. In 11 of the 14 cases (78.6%), the interviewers were able to reach agreement on the presence of each specific sphere of worry, and to agree on the unrealistic or excessive nature of the worry. A kappa coefficient of .90 was obtained when calculated on the interviewers' ratings of the excessive/unrealistic nature of the 35 specific spheres of worry indentified in the 14 patients. Finally, in another study using the ADIS-R (but at a center other than CSAD), Borkovec et al. (see Chapter 2) examined the reliability of GAD patients' responses to the specific ADIS-R question "Do you worry excessively about minor things?" during two independent interviews. The results indicated that 80% of patients gave consistent responses to this question. This figure is low relative to agreement attained by raters, suggesting that clinical judgment of the excessive/unrealistic nature of patients' worry is more reliable than patients' self-reports.

Conclusions

The current evidence for the reliability of DSM-III-R GAD and some of its criteria is encouraging in some areas, although several questions need further study. Mannuzza et al. (1989) found good reliability for lifetime GAD, using only the DSM-III-R somatic symptoms; however, the poor reliability for current episodes of GAD stands in contrast to the fair reliability for full DSM-III-R current GAD obtained in the CSAD sample, as well as good reliability in this sample when a criterion of strict agreement on

GAD as a principal diagnosis only was dropped. Also in contrast with the Mannuzza et al. findings, the CSAD sample showed very good reliability of GAD in the presence of a mood disorder.

As noted above, excessive or unrealistic worry appears to be more easily identified than physical symptoms of anxiety, and may be a better discriminator of anxiety and depressive diagnoses; however, problems still remain with this, particularly if PDA accompanies GAD. At this point, additional studies are necessary to determine whether similar reliability can be obtained with other instruments at other centers, and we are examining the possibility of analyzing existing data sets to answer this question.

The evidence also suggests that interviewers can reliably identify the content of GAD worries, and can agree on whether the worry is excessive or unrealistic, although the term "unrealistic" presents problems since most patients consider their worries basically realistic. This puts more of a burden on the term "excessive." Preliminary evidence also indicates that there is consistency between structured interviews and self-monitoring instruments in the content of worry reported by patients. In view of these findings, it seems that DSM-III-R has correctly designated worry as an essential or defining feature of GAD. Experience would suggest that the following spheres might be listed in criterion A: family/home and inter-personal relationships; finances; work/school; illness/health/injury; and miscellaneous or routine daily activities. It would also seem that criterion A should indicate that the excessive or unrealistic nature of worry should be judged by the clinician, and should not be based solely on a patient's self-report.

In contrast to the reliability of ratings of worry, ratings of the physical symptoms of anxiety are generally poor. This poor reliability may be due to inconsistency in patients' reports of such specific symptoms. It is difficult to suggest possible changes on the basis of the available data from Fyer et al. (1989) and the CSAD sample, because no one symptom or set of symptoms showed good reliability across both studies. However, we have reported elsewhere (Benshoof, Moras, Di Nardo, & Barlow, 1991) that the DSM-III criteria of moderate symptomatology in three of the four general areas (motor tension, autonomic hyperactivity, apprehensive ex-pectation, vigilance and scanning) accurately discriminated GAD patients from patients with other anxiety disorders. Although this study did not assess the reliability of these ratings, the results suggest that it might be worthwhile to examine the utility of modifying criterion D in DSM-III-R so that it is similar to DSM-III. Agreement on this criterion would be defined as a match on the general areas, rather than on specific symptoms. Because apprehensive expectation is subsumed under criterion A of DSM-III-R GAD, there would be three general areas (motor tension, autonomic hyperactivity, and vigilance and scanning), and the diagnosis would require symptomatology in two areas. Specific symptoms could still be retained as descriptors, but not required. Another option, perhaps a more viable and specific one, is described below.

In this section, we have left aside questions of the discriminative power of the specific criteria for GAD. Of course, it is necessary to establish the reliability of the criteria before determining whether the criteria can distinguish GAD patients from those with other Axis I disorders and from normals. There is now good evidence for the reliability of ratings of excessive worry, and we have already reviewed evidence that patients with GAD differ from normals in the excessiveness of worry and in the number of spheres of worry. The next step is to determine whether these dimensions discriminate GAD from other anxiety disorders and from mood disorders. The investigation of symptoms that discriminate GAD from dysthymia is particularly important, in view of the DSM-IV Anxiety Disorders Workgroup's interest in considering a mixed anxiety–depression category in DSM-IV (see Chapters 7 and 8). The search for discriminative criteria should extend beyond the DSM-III-R criteria. For example, Sanderson and Barlow (1990) reported that a question from the ADIS-R ("Do you worry excessively about minor things?") had a positive predictive power of .36 and a negative predictive power of .96 (see also Chapter 2). This means that a positive response to this question does not necessarily confirm the GAD diagnosis, but a negative response almost certainly rules out GAD. At the CSAD, we are currently examining the discriminative power of this and other criteria on a larger sample of patients.

LOOKING AHEAD TO DSM-IV

Despite the relatively brief period of time since the appearance of DSM-III-R, the process leading to DSM-IV (and ICD-10) is well underway. Reasons for this relative haste, as well as the empirically based process used to arrive at DSM-IV criteria, have been outlined elsewhere (Widiger, Frances, Pincus, Davis, & First, in press). To summarize briefly, the DSM-IV Anxiety Disorders Workgroup has been divided into subgroups examining each of the DSM-III-R anxiety disorders. These subgroups in turn commissioned a variety of review papers on the criteria and undertook to reanalyze existing data sets that might not as yet be in the public domain, if these data sets had a bearing on DSM-IV criteria. On the basis of these reviews and reanalyses, criteria were developed that will now be subjected to field trials (in many instances) to test their reliability and validity, pursuant to publication of DSM-IV in early 1993. During the early spring of 1991, as this chapter was in preparation, new criteria for DSM-IV GAD had been formulated. It is unlikely that these criteria will constitute the final word, since they are subject to data from subsequent field trials and to further deliberations by the Anxiety Disorders Workgroup, as well as the DSM-IV Task Force. Nevertheless, it is informative in terms of the development of the DSM-IV criteria to look at progress to this point.

Before we list the criteria themselves, it is important to review the major deficiencies that recent data have elucidated in DSM-III-R criteria. First, overall kappa coefficients are not as good as those for some other anxiety disorders, such as OCD or social phobia. Of course, one fundamental difference between GAD and some other anxiety diagnoses is that these other diagnoses are often characterized by an outstanding key feature— one that is easily differentiated from features of other anxiety disorders, at least in its prototypical presentation. It is possible that the pervasive worry in GAD, which has come to be its key and defining feature, by its very nature intersects and overlaps with other anxiety disorders in a way that makes it inherently less discriminatory. On the other hand, it is possible that additional data will lead to sharper and more discriminating definitions. The fact is that "anxiety" (particularly in its somatic presentation, as exemplified by autonomic hyperactivity) is fundamentally a presenting characteristic of all anxiety disorders, with the possible exception of simple phobia. Barlow (1988) thus puts the burden on definitions of chronic worry for purposes of discriminant validity. Nevertheless, if one cannot identify associated somatic symptoms reliably, then this can only lead to lower kappa coefficients for the GAD diagnosis as a whole. Our analysis of sources of disagreement between raters attempting to identify DSM-III-R GAD points to identification of these somatic symptoms as the primary weakness. Criteria on chronic worry, on the other hand, seem reasonably satisfactory but may be subject to improvement, pending further analyses as suggested below.

Table 5.8 presents some of the proposed DSM-IV criteria for GAD, as proposed in the spring of 1991. These proposed criteria accomplish several purposes, based on collected data and literature reviews. Proposed criteria A, B, C, and D essentially split criterion A in DSM-III-R into smaller and more user-friendly components. After the temporal criteria are restated in A, the major qualifiers are stated in criteria B, C, and D. Specifically, "excessive" is now highlighted, since clinicians have found this criterion most useful in ascertaining the pathological nature of worry. "Unrealistic," on the other hand, has proven less useful, since most patients with GAD would judge their worries to be realistic (while agreeing that

TABLE 5.8. Proposed DSM-IV GAD Criteria Set (September 1990 Draft)

A. Unrealistic anxiety and worry (apprehensive expectations), more days than not, for a period of at least 6 months.

B. The worry is excessive (*i.e., intensity, frequency or distress generated by the worry is out of proportion to the likelihood or impact of the feared event*), and does not lead to corrective or constructive action.

C. The worry is pervasive (i.e., not focused on just one particular life circumstance).

D. *The person finds it difficult to control the worry and to focus attention on the tasks at hand.*

E. If another Axis I disorder is present, the focus of the anxiety and worry is unrelated to it, e.g., the anxiety or worry is not about having a panic attack (as in Panic Disorder), being embarrassed in public (as in Social Phobia), being contaminated (as in Obsessive Compulsive Disorder), gaining weight (as in Anorexia Nervosa), or having a serious illness (as in Hypochondriasis).

G. *The worry or associated somatic symptoms interfere with social or occupational functioning, or there is marked distress about having these worries or somatic symptoms.*

---

they might be excessive and uncontrollable), and clinicians then find themselves in a position of making this difficult judgment. For this reason, the term "unrealistic" may not be retained in future revisions.

Criterion C takes the place of the conservative tack of specifying two different spheres. This criterion captures more accurately the notion that these individuals are worried chronically and pervasively. The possibility that somebody may present with only one major sphere of worry and yet meet criteria for GAD would be mitigated by the necessity of meeting both criteria B and D, as well as the differential diagnosis presented in criterion E. The uncontrollability of the worry process, described in criterion D, has also emerged from recent data as a central component of pathological or chronic worry (see Chapter 2). In addition, "having a serious illness (as in Hypochondriasis)" has been added to criterion E, to help delineate the boundary with hypochondriasis—particularly in view of a current proposal to incorporate hypochondriasis into the anxiety disorders. Once again, there is no guarantee that this proposal will make it into DSM-IV (or even last through 1991, for that matter).

Regarding the somatic symptoms, further efforts are underway to reanalyze existing data or collect new data that might point to the best way to handle this issue, particularly in view of the marked unreliability of the current criterion D in DSM-III-R. The other difficulty is that the requirement of identifying 6 out of 18 symptoms is user-unfriendly and implies a degree of precision that simply does not exist. Therefore, one possible solution would be to substitute a more general statement that there should be associated symptoms of autonomic hyperactivity, motor tension, vigilance, and scanning, with examples given for each. This criterion might be strengthened a bit by adding criterion G (specifying impairment or distress), in order to ensure the clinical significance of the disturbance. This option would, of course, bring this particular criterion closer to the original DSM-III criterion.

Other options are possible. If one were to stick with a list of specific somatic symptoms (as in DSM-III-R), then ideally one would want to reduce the list to a more manageable, reliable, and internally consistent number of symptoms. Efforts are currently underway at the CSAD to see whether this can be achieved. Specifically, six somatic symptoms identified as possessing both reliability and discriminant validity are being evaluated. These are "tense," "restless," "easily fatigued," "keyed up or on the edge," "irritable," and "having difficulty concentrating." A seventh symptom, "sleep disturbance," is also being scrutinized. Furthermore, these symptoms would be used as examples of somatic manifestation of GAD in a question such as the following: "During the past 6 months, have you been feeling physically tense or nervous—by that, I mean restless, easily fatigued, keyed up or on edge, having difficulty concentrating, or irritable?" Severity would also be assessed. If the data indicate that this option works, it will be far more user-friendly.

In any case, the empirically based nature of DSM-IV will require that any substantial changes be data-based before implementation. Ascertaining the relative advantages of the proposed revisions in this manner is a task that lies ahead of us.

REFERENCES

American Psychiatric Association. (1980). *Diagnostic and statistical manual of mental disorders* (3rd ed.). Washington, DC: Author.

American Psychiatric Association. (1987). *Diagnostic and statistical manual of mental disorders* (3rd ed., rev.). Washington, DC: Author.

Barlow, D. H. (1987). The classification of anxiety disorders. In G. L. Tischler (Ed.), *Diagnosis and classification in psychiatry: A critical appraisal of DSM-III*. Cambridge, England: Cambridge University Press.

Barlow, D. H. (1988). *Anxiety and its disorders: The nature and treatment of anxiety and panic*. New York: Guilford Press.

Barlow, D. H., Blanchard, E. B., Vermilyea, J. A., Vermilyea, B. B., & Di Nardo, P. A. (1986). Generalized anxiety and generalized anxiety disorder: Description and reconceptualization. *American Journal of Psychiatry, 143*, 40–44.

Barlow, D. H., Di Nardo, P. A., Vermilyea, B. B., Vermilyea, J. A., & Blanchard, E. B. (1986). Co-morbidity and depression among the anxiety disorders: Issues in diagnosis and classification. *Journal of Nervous and Mental Disease*, *174*, 63–72.

Benshoof, B. B., Moras, K., Di Nardo, P. A., & Barlow, D. H. (1991). *An examination of key features of three anxiety disorders*. Manuscript in preparation.

Breslau, N., & Davis, G. C. (1985). DSM-III generalized anxiety disorder: An empirical investigation of more stringent criteria. *Psychiatry Research*, *143*, 231–238.

Craske, M. G., Rapee, R. M., Jackel, L., & Barlow, D. H. (1989). Qualitative dimensions of worry in DSM-III-R generalized anxiety disorder subjects and nonanxious controls. *Behaviour Research and Therapy*, *27*, 397–402.

Di Nardo, P. A., & Barlow, D. H. (1988). *Anxiety Disorders Interview Schedule—Revised (ADIS-R)*. Albany: Center for Stress and Anxiety Disorders, University at Albany, State University of New York.

Di Nardo, P. A., O'Brien, G. T., Barlow, D. H., Waddell, M. T., & Blanchard, E. B. (1983). Reliability of DSM-III anxiety disorder categories using a new structured interview. *Archives of General Psychiatry*, *40*, 1070–1075.

Fleiss, J. L., Nee, J. C. M., & Landis, J. R. (1979). Large sample variance of kappa in the case of different sets of raters. *Psychological Bulletin*, *86*, 974–977.

Fyer, A. J., Mannuzza, S., Martin, L. Y., Gallops, M. S., Endicott, J., Schleyer, B., Gorman, J. M., Liebowitz, M. R., & Klein, D. F. (1989). Reliability of anxiety assessment: II. Symptom agreement. *Archives of General Psychiatry*, *46*, 1102–1110.

Jablensky, A. (1985). Approaches to the definition and classification of anxiety and related disorders in European psychiatry. In A. H. Tuma & J. D. Maser (Eds.), *Anxiety and the anxiety disorders*. Hillsdale, NJ: Erlbaum.

Mannuzza, S., Fyer, A. J., Martin, M. S., Gallops, M. S., Endicott, J., Gorman, J., Liebowitz, M. R., & Klein, D. F. (1989). Reliability of anxiety assessment: I. Diagnostic agreement. *Archives of General Psychiatry*, *46*, 1093–1101.

Sanderson, W. C., & Barlow, D. H. (1990). A description of patients diagnosed with DSM-III-Revised generalized anxiety disorder. *Journal of Nervous and Mental Disease*, *178*, 588–591.

Widiger, T. A., Frances, A. J., Pincus, H. A., Davis, W., & First, M. (in press). Toward an empirical classification for DSM-IV. *Journal of Abnormal Psychology* [Special issue].

6

Chronic Anxiety and Generalized Anxiety Disorder: Issues in Comorbidity

WILLIAM C. SANDERSON
SCOTT WETZLER
Albert Einstein College of Medicine/Montefiore Medical Center

"Comorbidity" refers to the concurrent presence of independent psychological disorders. In instances of comorbidity, the patient meets diagnostic criteria for more than one syndrome, and is therefore assigned multiple diagnoses. These multiple diaganoses, taken together, account for the patient's entire clinical presentation, symptomatology, and course of illness.

Past classification systems, such as the third edition of the *Diagnostic and Statistical Manual of Mental Disorders* (DSM-III; American Psychiatric Association, 1980), impeded the identification of comorbid syndromes because they contained hierarchical exclusionary rules; for the most part, these prohibited the assignment of more than one Axis I diagnosis to a patient. In the DSM-III hierarchical system, certain diagnoses took precedence, and other diagnoses were subsumed under disorders that occupied a higher diagnostic status. When a patient presented with a heterogeneous clinical picture, all symptomatology was considered a manifestation of the principal disorder, and the patient was therefore assigned only one diagnosis. For example, since affective disorders occupied a higher position than anxiety disorders in the DSM-III, the presence of panic attacks did not require the diagnosis of panic disorder (PD) if the clinican judged that the panic attacks were "due to" major depression (MD). In fact, according to the DSM-III, the presence of MD generally excluded any of the anxiety disorders.

Although all anxiety disorders were assigned secondary status in the DSM-III, the DSM-III designated generalized anxiety disorder (GAD) as a residual category (as noted in Chapter 5), thereby placing it at the low end of the diagnostic hierarchy. The clinician was not permitted to make a diagnosis of GAD if the presenting anxiety was "due to another physical or mental disorder" (p. 232). Since chronic generalized anxiety is a prominent feature of many different psychological syndromes (e.g., MD, schizophrenia, bipolar disorder, dysthymia, and especially all of the other anxiety disorders), this rule excluded GAD from consideration as a comorbid diagnosis.

The hierarchical exclusion rules used in DSM-III artificially obscured the independence of anxiety disorders and of GAD in particular. Since there is, in fact, no empirical evidence that anxiety disorders are secondary to depressive disorders (e.g., Sanderson, Beck, & Beck, 1990), these exclusion rules were, for the most part, dropped in DSM-III-R. Clinicans are now allowed to give "multiple diagnoses when different syndromes occur together in one episode of illness" (American Psychiatric Association, 1987, p. xxiv). On the basis of their relative severity and interference with the patient's functioning, one of these multiple diagnoses is identified as the patient's "principal" disorder, although the other disorders are also accorded clinical significance. Thus, DSM-III-R recognizes the importance of comorbidity more fully than any prior diagnostic system has done, especially in regard to GAD.

In DSM-III-R, two substantial revisions were made that have influenced the comorbidity of GAD. GAD is no longer a "residual" diagnostic category, and therefore may now be diagnosed independently of and in addition to other mental disorders. At the same time, the diagnostic criteria for GAD have been further specified and made more stringent (see Chapter 5, this volume). On the one hand, eliminating the exclusion rule has meant that GAD is more frequently diagnosed (on its own and as a comorbid disorder). On the other hand, establishing conservative diagnostic criteria has meant that fewer patients meet these diagnostic criteria.

SIGNIFICANCE OF COMORBIDITY

Patterns of comorbidity have important clinical and scientific implications, and thus it is unfortunate that prior to DSM-III-R comorbid psychological diagnoses were, relatively speaking, ignored. In fact, comorbid diagnoses are very common (Boyd et al., 1984). Recent studies using DSM-III (without exclusion rules) and DSM-III-R criteria have shown that a majority of outpatients seeking treatment may be diagnosed with multiple Axis I disorders (Barlow, Di Nardo, Vermilyea, Vermilyea, & Blanchard, 1986; Di Nardo & Barlow, 1990; de Ruiter, Ruken, Garssen, van Schaik, &

Kraaimaat, 1989; Sanderson, Beck, & Beck, 1990; Sanderson, Di Nardo, Rapee, & Barlow, 1990; Wolf et al., 1988). These data are consistent with Boyd et al.'s (1984) initial finding that the presence of any psychiatric disorder increases the likelihood of having another disorder. It appears that when clinicians evaluate patients carefully, using structured interviews, they usually uncover multiple disorders. These studies support the changes made in DSM-III-R, which allow the clinician to diagnose multiple disorders to account for the full range of presenting symptomatology.

The practice of assigning a single diagnosis is in many cases inadequate to convey the overall level of psychopathology. By recognizing the presence of more than one disorder, the clinician is in a position to offer better, more comprehensive treatment. Conversely, by ignoring comorbid diagnoses, the clinician will offer less than optimal treatment. In our clinical experience, for example, patients with MD and GAD together are unable to tolerate the increased anxiety and agitation that occur during the early days of treatment with fluoxetine (Prozac). These patients require concomitant treatment with an anxiolytic medication, such as one of the benzodiazepines. Thus, by recognizing the presence of the associated anxiety syndrome from the outset, the clinician will offer more effective treatment and will engender better patient compliance with medications.

The course, prognosis, and treatment response for patients with multiple psychological disorders have been shown to differ from those of patients with a single disorder (Fyer, Liebowitz, & Klein, 1990). For example, a recent review paper found that patients with concurrent PD and MD exhibited a greater degree of psychopathology and did not respond as well to "conventional antidepressants" than did patients with MD alone (Grunhaus, 1988). In one study, relapse was much higher in the comorbid group during a 2-year follow-up (Coryell et al., 1988). Although comparable data regarding the course, prognosis, and treatment response of patients with MD and GAD have not yet been collected, a similar scenario may be envisioned. Having two disorders would be expected to be worse than suffering from just one.

Patterns of comorbidity have important scientific implications as well. For example, when two disorders, such as any of the anxiety and depressive disorders, typically co-occur, it may be thought that they have a common etiology or that a shared vulnerability predisposes the individual to both disorders. Alternatively, the etiology of comorbid disorders may be different from the etiology of any single disorder when it presents in isolation. That is, a patient with GAD and MD may have a different underlying pathology from that of a patient with either GAD or MD alone.

Patterns of comorbidity also provide information concerning the genetic transmission of psychiatric illnesses. For example, relatives of individuals with the comorbid pattern of MD and an anxiety disorder are at greater risk for developing one of these disorders than are relatives of individuals with MD without an anxiety disorder (Leckman, Merikangas, Pauls, Prusoff, & Weissman, 1983).

In summary, close attention should be paid to the diagnosis of multiple disorders. There are good clinical and scientific reasons to do so. Once a clinician or researcher identifies one psychological disorder, he or she should continue the assessment to ascertain the presence of other disorders. All current evidence suggests that comorbid mental disorders are quite frequent.

FREQUENCY OF COMORBIDITY

The best estimate of the comorbidity of GAD may be derived from epidemiological studies. Unfortunately, comorbidity data from the recent Epidemiologic Catchment Area study are not yet available concerning GAD (M. M. Weissman, personal communication, July 24, 1990), and therefore no conclusions may be drawn about the co-occurrence of GAD and other major disorders in the general population at the present time. A more skewed estimate may be obtained by examining patients who present for treatment, although this population is self-selected and may have more severe forms of the disorders (Sanderson & Barlow, 1990).

The comorbidity studies that have addressed this question have utilized vastly different diagnostic inclusion and exclusion criteria. For instance, Breslau and Davis (1985a, 1985b) used an early draft of the DSM-III-R criteria to diagnose GAD; this draft did not include the current criterion of two spheres of worry. In this review, we only consider those studies that have used narrow criteria similar to those of DSM-III-R. Were we to review studies with more liberal inclusion diagnostic criteria, or studies that excluded GAD as an independent disorder (i.e., those using DSM-III criteria), then differences in rates of comorbidity would merely reflect these differences in diagnostic practices. Thus, there are only four relevant studies to review (Barlow, Di Nardo, et al., 1986; de Ruiter et al., 1989; Di Nardo & Barlow, 1990; Sanderson, Di Nardo, et al., 1990), all of which evaluated a total of 74 GAD patients presenting for treatment at anxiety disorders clinics. Despite the small sample, the comorbidity findings suggest some interesting trends.

There are two ways to calculate the frequency of comorbidity of GAD: (1) What is the frequency of other psychological disorders when GAD is the principal diagnosis? and (2) What is the frequency of GAD when another psychological disorder is the principal diagnosis? In each of the studies, all patients were given a structured interview—the Anxiety Disorders

Interview Schedule—Revised (ADIS-R) or the Structured Clinical Interview for DSM-III-R (SCID)—that covers all DSM-III-R disorders. Comorbidity was defined as the presence of multiple current DSM-III-R disorders, and past disorders were disregarded.

Table 6.1 summarizes the findings for the frequency of comorbid diagnoses for patients with a principal diagnosis of GAD, and Table 6.2 summarizes the findings for the frequency of GAD as an additional diagnosis for patients with other psychological conditions. The most striking overall finding is that 68% (50 of 74; range, 45–91%) of patients with GAD had an additional disorder. The magnitude of this comorbidity may be appreciated by comparing it to rates of comorbidity of other anxiety disorders. In the same studies, 54% (307 of 565; range between studies, 46–66%) of patients with other anxiety disorders had an additional disorder (see Table 6.2 for the rate of comorbidity for each disorder). In general, GAD had higher comorbidity than these other disorders.

Only one study (Sanderson, Di Nardo, et al., 1990) made a statistical comparison of the comorbid patterns; it was found that simple and social phobias were the most prevalent disorders associated with GAD.

The frequency of GAD for patients with other syndromes is presented in Table 6.2. Overall, the frequency of GAD as a comorbid diagnosis was 14% (100 of 696; range between studies, 1–21%). A closer analysis of these data reveals that GAD was a comorbid diagnosis for 9% (36 of 402) of patients with the other anxiety disorders, and for 22% (64 of 294) of patients with the depressive disorders (i.e., MD and dysthymia). We can conclude that patients with depressive disorders are more likely to have GAD as well than are patients with anxiety disorders (see also Chapter 5, this volume).

In conclusion, the majority of patients with GAD receive comorbid diagnoses. Thus, when the clinician treats a patient with GAD, he or she should make certain to evaluate for other conditions as well.

Interestingly, the frequency of GAD as a comorbid syndrome (according to DSM-III-R criteria) is relatively rare, especially for other anxiety disorders. Although generalized anxiety may be a common component of many anxiety and depressive syndromes (Barlow, Blanchard, Vermilyea, Vermilyea, & Di Nardo, 1986), generalized anxiety *disorder* is not commonly associated with them. In a sense, these data vindicate the authors of the DSM-III-R, who redefined GAD as an independent syndrome rather than as a residual disorder. The rationale of DSM-III had been that GAD was a residual disorder because generalized anxiety is a feature of many different psychological syndromes. In fact, according to DSM-III-R criteria, the syndrome of GAD is not often assigned as an additional diagnosis to other conditions. Most surprising to us is the lack of association between GAD and other anxiety disorders.

TABLE 6.1. Comorbidity of DSM-III and DSM-III-R Disorders in Patients with a Principal Diagnosis of GAD

Study and diagnostic criteria	n	% with comorbidity	Comorbid (additional) diagnoses	Comments
Barlow, Di Nardo, Vermilyea, Vermilyea, & Blanchard (1986); DSM-III	12	83% (10/12)	42% simple phobia (5/12) 33% social phobia (4/12) 17% agoraphobia (2/12) 17% dysthymia (2/12)	Modified DSM-III hierarchical exclusion rules. Used diagnostic criteria for GAD that were similar to those in the DSM-III-R. Structured interview: ADIS.
de Ruiter, Ruken, Garssen, van Schaik, & Kraaimaat (1989); DSM-III-R	9	67% (6/9)	56% simple phobia (5/9) 33% dysthymia (3/9) 11% obsessive compulsive (1/9)	Structured interview: ADIS-R.
Di Nardo & Barlow (1990); DSM-III	31	45% (14/31)	29% simple phobia (9/31) 16% social phobia (5/31) 6% major depression (2/31) 6% dysthymia (2/31) 3% panic disorder (1/31) 3% obsessive compulsive (1/31)	Same as Barlow et al. (1986). Used a severity threshold—counted only those diagnoses that reached "clinical severity" (i.e., required treatment).
Sanderson, Di Nardo, Rapee, & Barlow (1990); DSM-III-R	22	91% (20/22)	59% social phobia (13/22) 27% panic disorders (6/22) 27% dysthymia (6/22) 23% simple phobia (5/22) 14% major depression (3/22) 9% obsessive compulsive (2/22)	Structured interview: ADIS-R.

Note. Patients were eligible to receive more than one comorbid diagnosis.

TABLE 6.2. Percentage of Patients Receiving GAD as a Comorbid Diagnosis

Study	Principal diagnosis	% receiving any comorbid diagnosis	% receiving GAD as comorbid diagnosis
Barlow, Di Nardo, et al. (1986)	Agoraphobia	51% (21/41)	2% (1/41)
	Social phobia	47% (9/19)	5% (1/19)
	Panic disorder	88% (15/17)	0% (0/17)
	Simple phobia	57% (4/7)	0% (0/7)
	Obsessive compulsive	100% (6/6)	17% (1/6)
	Major depression	100% (6/6)	17% (1/6)
	Overall	64% (61/96)	4% (4/96)
de Ruiter et al. (1989)	PDA	59% (23/56)	0% (0/56)
	Panic disorder	65% (11/17)	0% (0/17)
	Major depression	100% (8/8)	0% (0/8)
	Dysthymia	88% (7/8)	12% (1/8)
	Simple phobia	0% (0/3)	0% (0/3)
	Social phobia	67% (2/3)	0% (0/3)
	Obsessive compulsive	33% (1/3)	0% (0/3)
	Agoraphobia w/out panic	100% (3/3)	0% (0/3)
	Overall	54% (55/101)	1% (1/101)
Di Nardo & Barlow (1990)	Agoraphobia	45% (39/86)	7% (6/86)
	Panic disorder	46% (31/67)	16% (11/67)
	Social phobia	42% (20/48)	4% (2/48)
	Simple phobia	33% (8/24)	8% (2/24)
	Obsessive compulsive	47% (7/15)	13% (2/15)
	Major depression	73% (8/11)	45% (5/11)
	Dysthymia	78% (7/9)	33% (3/9)
	Overall	46% (120/260)	8% (21/260)

(continued)

125

TABLE 6.2. (*Continued*)

Study	Principal diagnosis	% receiving any comorbid diagnosis	% receiving GAD as comorbid diagnosis
Sanderson, Di Nardo, et al. (1990)	PDA	69% (38/55)	13% (7/55)
	Social phobia	58% (14/24)	8% (2/24)
	Simple phobia	53% (9/17)	6% (1/17)
	Obsessive compulsive	83% (10/12)	0% (0/12)
	Overall	66% (71/108)	9% (10/108)
Sanderson, Beck, & Beck (1990)	Major depression	65% (128/197)	20% (40/197)
	Dysthymia	67% (42/63)	22% (14/63)
	Overall	65% (170/260)	21% (54/260)

Note. PDA, panic disorder with agoraphobia.

CHRONIC ANXIETY AS A DIMENSION OF PSYCHOPATHOLOGY

As noted above, "comorbidity" typically refers to the co-occurrence of multiple syndromes or disorders. This way of thinking derives from the "medical model," in which psychiatric syndromes are considered whole entities with distinct configurations of characteristics qualitatively different from each other, which appear and disappear as whole entities (Katz & Wetzler, in press). The unit of classification, therefore, is the disorder itself. This categorical or holistic model permits the easy determination of comorbidity, since a disorder is either present or absent.

An alternative way of thinking about comorbidity is the dimensional or componential approach to psychopathology. In this view, all psychopathology consists of components (e.g., anxiety, hostility, depression) that may be conceived of as independent or partially so, and thus should be considered as separate factors in themselves (Katz & Wetzler, in press). The components in this approach represent the building blocks of psychopathology, rather than the overarching disorder itself.

The componential approach, for example, considers chronic and generalized anxiety to be an essential feature of almost all kinds of psychopathology (Wetzler & Katz, 1989). It may be found most obviously in GAD and other anxiety disorders, but it is present to a large degree in MD, bipolar disorder, schizophrenia, substance abuse, and many other disorders. It is a dimension of psychopathology that exists to a greater or lesser extent in the description, characterization, and measurement of any disorder. As such, it makes sense to consider the comorbidity of generalized anxiety as a dimension of many different syndromes, not just the comorbidity of GAD as a disorder.

Although our review indicates that GAD is rarely assigned as a comorbid disorder, generalized anxiety is both a commonplace and important aspect of all psychopathology (Barlow, Blanchard, et al., 1986). Therefore, using a categorical diagnostic system (e.g., DSM-III-R) underestimates the prevalence of generalized anxiety as a dimension.

It is impossible to obtain an accurate estimate of the prevalence of generalized anxiety as a comorbid dimension, because it is inextricably entangled with other dimensions of psychopathology. For example, in MD, the components of anxiety and depression are linked together and "merge insensibly" with each other (Lewis, 1934). These two components of psychopathology bear such a marked resemblance to each other that the process of separating them is an abstract procedure requiring sophisticated statistical analysis (i.e., factor analysis). Anxiety and depression rarely exist as "pure" entities; in almost all instances, they co-occur. Nonetheless, the differentiation of dimensions of anxiety and depression is possible, and provides important scientific and clinical information about the process of recovery from MD and about brain–behavior relationships (Wetzler & Katz, 1989). (See also Chapters 7 and 8 of this volume for an extended discussion on differentiating anxiety and depression.)

Generalized anxiety is such a prominent component of MD that MD patients score as highly on standardized scales of anxiety as they do on depression scales (Katz, Wetzler, Koslow, & Secunda, 1989; Wetzler, Kahn, Cahn, van Praag, & Asnis, 1990; Wetzler, Kahn, Strauman, & Dubro, 1989; see also Chapter 1, this volume). In addition, patients with MD and dysthymia have higher scores on anxiety scales than do patients with GAD and other anxiety disorders (Di Nardo & Barlow, 1990). Generalized anxiety is also present at high levels in bipolar disorder (Katz et al., 1984), schizophrenia (Katz et al., 1984; Katz, Marsella, & Dube, 1988), alcohol and drug problems (Kushner, Sher, & Beitman, 1990; Ross, Glaser, & Germanson, 1988), bulimia (Fairburn & Cooper, 1982), somatoform disorders (Adler, 1989), and psychophysiological disorders (Adler, 1989; Blanchard, Scharff, Schwarz, Suls, & Barlow, 1989).

The recognition of generalized anxiety as a frequent comorbid dimension of psychopathology is of great significance. This feature, which cuts across many different diagnostic categories, may in itself require independent consideration and treatment. Despite vast differences in the treatment of different disorders, the treatment of generalized anxiety within each disorder may remain fairly constant and must be attended to. For example, patients with alcohol dependence require independent treatment for the associated generalized anxiety. Thus, the clinician may choose to offer the alcoholic patient a conventional treatment similar to ones offered to GAD patients. To fail to do so would increase the likelihood of later relapse.

In conclusion, a dimensional or componential approach to under-standing the comorbidity of generalized anxiety offers a way of thinking that the traditional or categorical approach does not. It does not make arbitrary, all-or-nothing distinctions regarding the presence of generalized anxiety, and thus it highlights this omnipresent feature of psychopathology. As the clinician begins to appreciate when and where generalized anxiety is present, he or she will be able to offer a more comprehensive treatment.

COMORBIDITY OF GAD AND PERSONALITY DISORDERS

In our discussion of the comorbidity of GAD, we have thus far ignored the issue of the comorbidity of GAD and the various personality disorders.

To date, we are unaware of any published studies examining the frequency of personality disorders in GAD patients. This omission may be due in part to two related factors. First, both GAD and personality disorders have been overlooked as important diagnostic categories, and thus have received little research attention (Widiger & Rogers, 1989). Second, both GAD and personality disorders have been considered unreliable diagnostic entities with fuzzy diagnostic criteria (Mannuzza et al., 1989; Frances, 1982; see Chapter 5, this volume). Until their diagnostic reliability improves and they receive the research attention they deserve, we may only speculate about the comorbidity of these disorders.

Our speculations are based in part on unpublished data collected at the Center for Cognitive Therapy, University of Pennsylvania School of Medicine (Sanderson & Beck, 1990). Thirty-two patients with a principal diagnosis of GAD were evaluated, using the section of the SCID for Axis II disorders (Spitzer, Williams, & Gibbons, 1987), prior to treatment. Sixteen (50%) of these patients were diagnosed with a comorbid personality disorder. The most common diagnoses were avoidant (5 of 32; 16%), dependent (4 of 32; 13%), and not otherwise specified (4 of 32; 13%). Other personality disorder diagnoses were paranoid (1 of 32; 3%), obsessive compulsive (1 of 32; 3%), and histrionic (1 of 32; 3%).

That there is substantial comorbidity of GAD and certain personality disorders is not surprising, although they are never listed as differential diagnostic alternatives in DSM-III-R. In particular, patients with GAD would be expected to exhibit characteristics of personality disorders within the anxious/fearful cluster (i.e., avoidant, dependent, obsessive compulsive, passive aggressive). The greatest overlap may be found between avoidant personality disorder and GAD, since fearfulness of social contact is a core component of both disorders. Avoidant personality disorder patients have a significant degree of generalized anxiety, and GAD patients are frequently hypersensitive to rejection and thus avoidant of many social interactions (Rapee, Sanderson, & Barlow, 1988). Similarly, we would expect some overlap between dependent personality disorder and GAD, since again fearfulness is a predominant feature of both. For example, a majority of patients with another anxiety disorder (i.e., panic disorder) have comorbid avoidant and dependent personality disorders (Reich & Noyes, 1987; Mavissakalian & Hamman, 1986).

In contrast to the anxious/fearful cluster of personality disorders, it is unlikely that GAD would be associated with certain other personality disorders, such as the anxiety-free antisocial personality disorder. However, there may be some relationship between GAD and histrionic personality disorder (i.e., excessive emotionality and seeking of reassurance regarding anxiety-laden issues) or paranoid personality disorder (i.e., suspiciousness at times of heightened anxiety). Further research is needed to clarify this important topic.

As is true for all Axis I–Axis II interactions, the presence of a comorbid personality disorder associated with GAD will influence the clinical presentation and psychotherapeutic treatment of the anxiety syndrome. For example, in our clinical experience, a GAD patient with dependent personality disorder is strikingly different from a GAD patient with borderline personality disorder. The dependent patient is clingy, submissive, and constantly seeking reassurance. This patient's anxiety is often triggered by dependency conflicts, such as a threat to his or her security. In contrast, the borderline patient is more chaotic, with tumultuous interpersonal relationships. The borderline patient's anxiety is often triggered by his or her identity disturbance, which then leads to hostility within relationships. Thus, psychotherapeutic tactics must take into account the characterological profile of the GAD patient.

GAD AS A PERSONALITY DISORDER

The separation of psychiatric disorders into two axes in DSM-III and DSM-III-R represents a major conceptual shift in diagnostic procedures. This distinction was based on the belief that personality disorders (coded on Axis II) are qualitatively different from all other syndromes (coded on Axis I). The primary difference between Axis I and Axis II has to do with the chronicity of the disorder. Personality disorders reflect "characteristic features [that] are typical of the person's long term functioning" (American Psychiatric Association, 1987, p. 335). They are believed to begin in "childhood or adolescence and persist in a stable form (without periods of remission or exacerbation) into adult life" (American Psychiatric Association, 1987, p. 16).

In contrast, Axis I disorders are believed to occur as discrete, obvious episodes that are not characteristic of the individual's long-standing functioning. There are remissions and exacerbations, and the age of onset of Axis I conditions may be much later than that for Axis II conditions. Essentially, Axis I disorders represent maladaptive *states* (i.e., the patient's transient symptomatology), and Axis II disorders represent maladaptive *traits* (i.e., features of the patient's enduring personality pattern) (Millon, 1981).

Axis I disorders are clear-cut manifestations of psychopathology, whereas Axis II disorders are not always distinct from normal functioning. For example, severe depression, psychosis, or PD is obviously pathological. Generally speaking, however, the behaviors exhibited by patients with personality disorders are not all that different from normal personality styles. Personality traits are characteristics that are distributed along a continuum in the entire population. Only those individuals on the extremes of the continuum will be considered pathological and diagnosed with a personality disorder (Millon, 1981; Frances, 1980). This is what is meant by a maladaptive personality trait (i.e., it interferes with the individual's long-standing social and/or occupational functioning).

Insofar as Axis II personality disorders are conceived as chronic patterns of maladaptive behavior that are not easily distinguishable from normal behavior, then we propose that GAD may best be considered a form of personality disorder as well. Typically, GAD patients present with a lifelong and chronic history of anxiety, apprehension, and somatic arousal (Anderson, Noyes, & Crowe, 1984; Barlow, Blanchard, et al., 1986; Cameron, Thyer, Nesse, & Curtis, 1986; Noyes, Clarkson, Crowe, Yates, & McChesney, 1987; Sanderson & Barlow, 1990). In many cases, there is no clear point of onset, or the onset dates from early adolescence. Thus, generalized anxiety appears to be trait-related, not state-related—a characteristic of an individual's long-standing personality.

Generalized anxiety also fulfills the second criterion of a personality disorder: It is a common feature of normal behavior. Everyone experiences anxiety and worry, unlike panic attacks, compulsions, or psychotic symptoms, which are limited to a much smaller segment of the population. Generalized anxiety is a basic psychological dimension that is present in everyone to a greater or lesser degree. For this reason, it is not easy to differentiate normal from pathological generalized anxiety (see Chapter 2, this volume; Craske, Rapee, Jackel, & Barlow, 1989). To do so, the clinician must take into account the impairment of the individual's social and occupational functioning. When the anxiety is sufficiently pervasive and impairs normal functioning, then a diagnosis of GAD is made. Clearly, this is a fairly subjective determination, as is the determination of the presence or absence of certain personality dimensions.

Since GAD more closely resembles a personality disorder than an Axis I syndrome, we support Akiskal's (1985) recommendation to modify and include "anxious personality disorder" among the Axis II disorders. Criteria should include the following, among others: (1) persistent, excessive worry about future circumstances (catastrophic thinking); (2) ruminations about past events; (3) somatic complaints; (4) marked feelings of tension and inability to relax; and (5) excessive concern about performance, achievement, and competence.

Including anxious personality disorder on Axis II would increase the consistency of the Axis I–Axis II (state–trait) distinction. If empirical evidence were to suggest that some GAD patients actually have an acute, transient course of generalized anxiety, then a separate GAD diagnostic category on Axis I would be warranted.

SUMMARY

The study of the comorbidity of GAD has been limited by the exclusionary rules used in prior classification systems. According to DSM-III-R criteria (in which GAD is no longer a "residual" category), it appears that the majority of the GAD patients receive comorbid diagnoses, especially simple and social phobias. Despite the prevalence of generalized anxiety across all disorders, GAD is rarely assigned as a comorbid diagnosis to patients with other anxiety disorders and is more frequently assigned to patients with depressive disorders. Although empirical data are nonexistent, it is our impression that there is substantial comorbidity between GAD and personality disorders, especially within the anxious/fearful cluster of personality disorders. In fact, certain lines of evidence suggest that GAD may be more appropriately considered as a personality disorder.

In conclusion, the observed pattern of comorbidity of GAD highlights the necessity of diagnosing multiple psychological disorders in a single patient.

REFERENCES

Adler, C. M. (1989). *Somatic and anxiety sensitivities: An investigation of the phenomenological relationships between somatoform anxiety and psychophysiological disorders*. Unpublished doctoral dissertation, University at Albany, State University of New York.

Akiskal, H. S. (1985). Anxiety: Definition, relationship to depression and proposal for an integrative model. In A. H. Tuma & J. D. Maser (Eds.), *Anxiety and the anxiety disorders*. Hillsdale, NJ: Erlbaum.

American Psychiatric Association. (1980). *Diagnostic and statistical manual of mental disorders* (3rd ed.). Washington, DC: Author.

American Psychiatric Association. (1987). *Diagnostic and statistical manual of mental disorders* (3rd ed., rev.). Washington, DC: Author.

Anderson, D. J., Noyes, R., & Crowe, R. R. (1984). A comparison of panic disorder and generalized anxiety disorder. *American Journal of Psychiatry, 141*, 572–575.

Barlow, D. H., Blanchard, E. B., Vermilyea, J. A., Vermilyea, B. B., & Di Nardo, P. A. (1986). Generalized anxiety and generalized anxiety disorder: Description and reconceptualization. *American Journal of Psychiatry, 143*, 40–44.

Barlow, D. H., Di Nardo, P. A., Vermilyea, B. B., Vermilyea, J. A., & Blanchard, E. B. (1986). Co-morbidity and depression among the anxiety disorders: Issues in classification and diagnosis. *Journal of Nervous and Mental Disease, 174*, 63–72.

Blanchard, E. B., Scharff, L., Schwarz, S. P., Suls, J. M., & Barlow, D. H. (1989). *The role of anxiety and depression in the irritable bowel syndrome.* Manuscript submitted for publication.

Boyd, J. H., Burke, J. D., Gruenberg, E., Holzer, C. E., Rae, D. S., George, L. K., Karno, M., Stoltzman, R., McEvoy, L., Nestadt, G. (1984). Exclusion criteria of DSM-III. *Archives of General Psychiatry, 41*, 983–989.

Breslau, N., & Davis, G. (1985a). DSM-III generalized anxiety disorder: An empirical investigation of more stringent criteria. *Psychiatry Research, 14*, 231–238.

Breslau, N., & Davis, G. C. (1985b). Further evidence on the doubtful validity of generalized anxiety disorder. *Psychiatry Research, 16*, 177–179.

Cameron, O. G., Thyer, B. A., Nesse, R. M., & Curtis, G. M. (1986). Symptom profiles of patients with DSM-III anxiety disorders. *American Journal of Psychiatry, 143*, 1132–1137.

Coryell, W., Endicott, J., Andreasen, N. C., Keller, M. B., Clayton, P. J., & Hirschfeld, R. M. A. (1988). Depression and panic attacks: The significance of overlap as reflected in follow-up and family study data. *American Journal of Psychiatry, 145*, 1138–1140.

Craske, M. G., Rapee, R. M., Jackel, L., & Barlow, D. H. (1989). Qualitative dimensions of worry in DSM-III-R generalized anxiety disorder subjects and nonanxious controls. *Behaviour Research and Therapy, 27*, 397–402.

de Ruiter, C., Ruken, H., Garssen, B., van Schaik, A., & Kraaimaat, F. (1989). Comorbidity among the anxiety disorders. *Journal of Anxiety Disorders, 3*, 57–68.

Di Nardo, P. A., & Barlow, D. H. (1990). Syndrome and symptom co-morbidity in the anxiety disorders. In J. D. Maser & C. R. Cloninger (Eds.), *Comorbidity in anxiety and mood disorders*. Washington, DC: American Psychiatric Press.

Frances, A. (1980). The DSM-III personality disorders section: A commentary. *American Journal of Psychiatry*, 1050–1054.

Frances, A. (1982). Categorical and dimensional systems of personality diagnosis: A comparison. *Comprehensive Psychiatry, 23*, 516–527.

Fyer, A. J., Liebowitz, M. R., & Klein, D. F. (1990). Treatment trials, co-morbidity, and syndromal complexity. In J. D. Maser & C. R. Cloninger (Eds.), *Comorbidity in anxiety and mood disorders*. Washington, DC: American Psychiatric Press.

Grunhaus, L. (1988). Clinical and psychobiological characteristics of simultaneous panic disorder and major depression. *American Journal of Psychiatry, 145*, 1214–1221.

Katz, M. M., Koslow, S., Berman, N., Secunda, S., Maas, J. W., Casper, R., Kocsis, J., & Stokes, P. (1984). A multi-vantaged approach to measurement of behavioral and affect states for clinical and psychobiological research. *Psychological Reports, 55* (Monograph Suppl.), 619–671.

Katz, M. M., Marsella, A., & Dube, K. C. (1988). On the expression of psychosis in different cultures: Schizophrenia in an Indian and a Nigerian community. *Culture, Medicine, and Psychiatry*, *12*, 331–355.

Katz, M. M., & Wetzler, S. (in press). Behavior measurement in psychobiological research. In *Encyclopedia of human biology* (Vol. 1). San Diego: Academic Press.

Katz, M. M., Wetzler, S., Koslow, S., & Secunda, S. (1989). Video methodology in the study of the psychopathology and treatment of depression. *Psychiatric Annals*, *19*, 372–381.

Kushner, M. G., Sher, K. J., & Beitman, B. D. (1990). The relation between alcohol problems and the anxiety disorders. *American Journal of Psychiatry*, *147*, 685–695.

Leckman, J. F., Merikangas, K. R., Pauls, D. L., Prusoff, B. A., & Weissman, M. M. (1983). Anxiety disorders and depression: Contradictions between family study data and DSM-III conventions. *American Journal of Psychiatry*, *140*, 880–882.

Lewis, A. (1934). Melancholia: A clinical survey of depressive states. *Journal of Mental Science*, *80*, 1–42.

Mannuzza, S., Fyer, A. J., Martin, L. Y., Gallops, M. S., Endicott, J., Gorman, J., Liebowitz, M. R., & Klein, D. F. (1989). Reliability of anxiety assessment: I. Diagnostic agreement. *Archives of General Psychiatry*, *46*, 1093–1101.

Mavissakalian, M., & Hamman, M. S. (1986). DSM-III personality disorders in agoraphobia. *Comprehensive Psychiatry*, *27*, 471–479.

Millon, T. (1981). *Disorders of personality*. New York: Wiley.

Noyes, R., Clarkson, C., Crowe, R. R., Yates, W. R., & McChesney, C. M. (1987). A family study of generalized anxiety disorder. *American Journal of Psychiatry*, *144*, 1019–1024.

Rapee, R. M., Sanderson, W. C., & Barlow, D. H. (1988). Social phobia features across the DSM-III-R anxiety disorders. *Journal of Psychopathology and Behavioral Assessment*, *10*, 287–299.

Reich, J. H., & Noyes, R. (1987). A comparison of DSM-III personality disorders in acutely ill panic and depressed patients. *Journal of Anxiety Disorders*, *1*, 123–131.

Ross, H. E., Glaser, F. B., & Germanson, T. (1988). The prevalence of psychiatric disorders in patients with alcohol and other drug problems. *Archives of General Psychiatry*, *45*, 1023–1031.

Sanderson, W. C., & Barlow, D.H. (1990). A description of patients diagnosed with DSM-III-Revised generalized anxiety disorder. *Journal of Nervous and Mental Disease*, *178*, 588–591.

Sanderson, W. C., & Beck, A. T. (1990). *Cognitive therapy for generalized anxiety disorder: A naturalistic study*. Manuscript submitted for publication.

Sanderson, W. C., Beck, A. T., & Beck, J. (1990). Syndrome comorbidity in patients with major depression or dysthymia: Prevalence and temporal relationships. *American Journal of Psychiatry*, *147*, 1025–1028.

Sanderson, W. C., Di Nardo, P. A., Rapee, R. M., & Barlow, D. H. (1990). Syndrome comorbidity in patients diagnosed with a DSM-III-R anxiety disorder. *Journal of Abnormal Psychology, 99,* 308–312.

Spitzer, R. L., Williams, J. B. W., & Gibbon, M. (1987). *Structured Clinical Interview for DSM-III-R (SCID)*. New York: Biometrics Research Department, New York State Psychiatric Institute.

Wetzler, S., Kahn, R. S., Cahn, W., van Praag, H. M., & Asnis, G. (1990). Psychological test characteristics of depressed and panic patients. *Psychiatry Research, 31,* 179–192.

Wetzler, S., Kahn, R., Strauman, T., & DuBro, A. (1989). The diagnosis of major depression by self-report. *Journal of Personality Assessment, 53,* 22–30.

Wetzler, S., & Katz, M. M. (1989). Problems with the differentiation of anxiety and depression. *Journal of Psychiatry Research, 23,* 1–12.

Widiger, T. A., & Rogers, J. H. (1989). Prevalence and comorbidity of personality disorders. *Psychiatric Annals, 19,* 132–136.

Wolf, A. S., Schubert, D. S. P., Patterson, M. B., Grande, T. P., Brocco, K. J., & Pendleton, L. (1988). Associations among major psychiatric diagnoses. *Journal of Consulting and Clinical Psychology, 56,* 292–294.

7

Mixed Anxiety–Depression: A New Diagnostic Category?

RICHARD E. ZINBARG
DAVID H. BARLOW
University at Albany, State University of New York

T he existing literature suggests that there are many patients with "mixed anxiety–depression" (MAD) or anxious or depressed symptoms alone that do not meet current definitional thresholds for *Diagnostic and Statistical Manual of Mental Disorders*, third edition, revised (DSM-III-R; American Psychiatric Assocation, 1987) Axis I anxiety and mood disorders; nonetheless, these patients show substantial impairment. They may present differently from patients with current Axis I anxiety and depressive disorders, and perhaps require different treatment (e.g., Klerman, 1989; Katon & Roy-Byrne, 1990; Clark & Watson, 1990; Barrett, Barrett, Oxman, & Gerber, 1988). Currently these individuals are poorly identified and inconsistently treated, and they evidently impose a substantial burden on the health care system. It is also noteworthy that patients presenting with DSM-III-R subdefinitional thresholds of anxiety and/or depressive symptoms seem to appear frequently in primary care settings. These observations, which are common around the world, have prompted the inclusion of a category of MAD (without criteria) in the most recent version of the *International Classification of Diseases* (ICD-10). Similarly, at the time of this writing (late 1990), the DSM-IV Task Force is considering the possible inclusion of a diagnostic category of MAD in DSM-IV.

In this chapter, we first provide an overview of recent studies examining conceptual, psychometric, and clinical aspects of the presentation of mixed anxious and depressive symptoms. We then describe an ongoing field trial whose purpose is to examine the feasibility and usefulness of creating a category of MAD for DSM-IV. As noted above, the category, if created, would include only those individuals who do not meet criteria for other DSM Axis I anxiety or depressive disorders. In other words, someone presenting with generalized anxiety disorder with accompanying depressive features such as anhedonia would not qualify. Similarly, someone presenting with comorbid diagnoses of an anxiety disorder and a depressive disorder would not qualify.

More importantly, from a conceptual point of view, consideration of the presentation of mixed anxiety and depressed features raises questions regarding the fundamental nature of chronic anxiety and depression and their relationship (see also Chapter 8). One possible model of this relationship has been outlined in Chapter 1. Specifically, MAD and its fundamental component, negative affect, may be the common cognitive–affective state priming the more specific features that currently define Axis I anxiety and depressive disorders. Examples of such features may be panic attacks, intrusive thoughts, or suicidal ideation.

PSYCHOMETRIC AND CONCEPTUAL ISSUES

A review of the relevant psychometric data by Clark and Watson (1990) addressed the issue of whether sufficient empirical evidence exists to warrant the inclusion of a MAD diagnosis in DSM-IV. To construct a conceptual framework regarding the relationship between depression and anxiety within which to address this question, they examined indices of the convergent and discriminant validity of measures of anxiety and depression (both self-report and clinical ratings) and factor-analytic studies of symptoms. They concluded that the evidence is consistent with a tripartite model of the relationship between anxiety and depression. This tripartite model is an elaboration of Tellegen's (1985) earlier work on negative and positive affect. The three elements of the tripartite model are negative affect or nonspecific general distress, features specific to anxiety, and features specific to depression.

The general-distress factor posited by Clark and Watson accounts for the fact that moderate to high correlations are consistently found between symptom measures of anxiety and depression. The second factor, containing features specific to anxiety, consists of physiological symptoms of hyperarousal that consistently tend to distinguish anxious and depressed diagnostic groups. The third factor, which is posited to be specific to depression, is lack of positive affect. Symptoms that indicate lack of positive affect are those associated with pervasive anhedonia, such as loss of interest/pleasure, apathy, hopelessness, and fatigue.

The question of how these three factors are combined in individuals remains unanswered. Are anxiety and depression entities that share sufficient symptoms to produce the strong observed correlations between them, yet whose specific components differentiate them sufficiently to define them as distinct syndromes? Or have attempts to differentiate anxiety and depression failed in part because there are sizeable groups of patients who cannot be meaningfully categorized simply as either anxious or depressed, because they either exhibit a wide variety of both types of specific symptoms, or else show primarily nonspecific symptoms? Clark and Watson concluded that the weight of the data suggests the latter.

Clark and Watson (1990) offered several recommendations for revisions of the DSM-III-R nomenclature that would affect the anxiety and mood disorder categories. These recommendations are based on the following rationale. Elevated levels of the nonspecific general-distress component of affective syndromes will nearly always be evident in anxious or depressed patients. Nonspecific general distress essentially signals the presence of the disorders. Therefore, the presence of a high level of negative affect suggests the relevance of anxiety and depressive diagnoses (and perhaps other diagnoses as well), but in and of itself offers no basis for finer discrimination. The two specific factors (i.e., physiological tension and pervasive anhedonia) provide an appropriate basis for the needed discrimination.

In regard to a possible category of MAD, Clark and Watson (1990) have suggested that many patients will show low levels of both specific factors; that is, neither marked physiological symptoms nor anhedonia will be particularly salient aspects of their symptom presentation. Such patients' predominant symptoms will therefore be nonspecific (e.g., distress, demoralization, irritability, mild disturbances of sleep and appetite, distractibility, vague somatic complaints), according to the tripartite model. For such patients, the development of a new diagnostic category has been recommended; this could be labeled MAD or perhaps "generalized mood disorder." Patients with the diagnosis would probably be most prevalent in general medical populations, but would not be uncommon in psychiatric settings.

CLINICAL FINDINGS

Recently, Katon and Roy-Byrne (1990) reviewed the clinical literature on MAD from community, primary care, and psychiatric samples. They concluded that the evidence strongly suggests the existence of a subgroup of people who have mixed anxiety and depressive symptoms, but who do not have enough symptoms of either type to meet criteria for existing DSM-III-R anxiety or mood disorders.

There is also considerable evidence suggesting that the incidence of comorbid anxious and depressive symptoms may be particularly prevalent in primary care settings. For example, Hiller, Zaudig, and Bose (1989) screened several hundred patients with a diagnostic checklist and found that the overlap between depressive and anxiety symptoms was much greater in the absence of an Axis I anxiety or mood disorder. More importantly, Katon and Roy-Byrne (1990) reviewed evidence suggesting that patients in primary care settings presenting with mixed anxiety and depressive symptoms are at risk of developing more severe mood or anxiety disorders after experiencing stressful life events. But before this happens, these patients somatize, present with significant impairment in their social and vocational roles, and utilize a disproportionate share of time in primary care settings. These findings point to the need to examine the prevalence of MAD, particularly in primary care settings.

Katon and Roy-Byrne (1990) also noted the prevalence of marked symptoms of anxiety and depression, sometimes referred to as "demoralization" (Dohrenwend, Shrout, Egri, & Mendelsohn, 1980), in community samples (e.g., Eaton, McCutcheon, Dryman, & Sorenson, in press). Barrett et al. (1988) assessed patients from a rural primary care practice for psychiatric disorder, using a modified Research Diagnostic Criteria (RDC) classification. By means of a structured interview, patients were evaluated for the following specific diagnostic conditions: minor depression; chronic intermittent minor depression; labile personality; generalized anxiety disorder; and a combined group consisting of panic and phobic states, masked/suspected depression, and MAD. The MAD group included individuals with symptoms of both anxiety and depression that were not of sufficient frequency or duration to meet the RDC requirements for a specific disorder. Overall, 26.5% of the 1,000 patients in the sample were thought to have a psychiatric disorder. The most common was masked/suspected depression (6.4%), followed by MAD (4.1%), episodic major or minor depression (4.1%), chronic intermittent depression or labile personality (3.9%), and generalized anxiety disorder (2.9%).

Several recent studies have addressed the issue of functional impairment associated with depressive symptoms that do not otherwise meet criteria for an Axis I disorder. For example, Wells et al. (1989) reported on the functional status and well-being of patients with depressive disorders, compared to a group of patients with depressive symptoms that did not meet criteria for a DSM-III mood disorder. The results indicated that patients with depressive symptoms that did not meet criteria for an Axis

I disorder were impaired in a number of areas, compared both to normal controls and to patients with chronic medical conditions. Depressive symptoms were associated with impairment in the areas of physical and social functioning, perceived current health, and role functioning at work and at home. Findings from this study also indicated that these patients had a substantial impact on the health care system. Because of the methodology in the study, anxiety symptoms were not assessed. However, in view of other data indicating a lack of differentiation between anxiety and depressive symptoms at this level (Hiller et al., 1989), it is possible that these patients also presented with symptoms of anxiety and could have been more accurately described as presenting with MAD. It should also be noted that this study did not control for the effects of a third variable (severity of medical illness) that could account for the relationship between depressive symptoms and impairment.

Broadhead, Blazer, George, and Kit Tse (1990) presented evidence from a prospective 1-year follow-up survey of a large community sample ($n = 2,980$) on functional impairment in three categories of depressive disorder. The depressive categories examined were as follows: (1) major depression, as defined by the Diagnostic Interview Schedule (DIS)/DSM-III criteria, and including double depression in the past 6 months; (2) dysthymia, as defined by the DIS/DSM-III criteria (lifetime diagnosis), but no copresent major depression; and (3) minor depression, as defined by having one or more symptoms of depression but not major depression or dysthymia during the past 6 months. Two indices of functional impairment were used: (1) number of work days missed within the past 3 months due to illness, and (2) number of disability days (i.e., person spent all or part of the day in bed, or was kept from usual activities because of feeling sick). Number of work days missed included number of times late to work, not just full days missed.

The three depressive groups were compared to an asymptomatic group (i.e., no DIS/DSM-III symptoms of depression during the 6 months prior to the interview) on the indices of functional impairment. Broadhead et al. (1990) presented several analyses, including frequencies and percentages of disability days and days missed, for the three depressed groups and the asymptomatic group. Odds ratios were computed for one or more disability days for the entire sample (i.e., employed and unemployed). For the group with minor depression, the risk of disability was 1.47 times more likely than for the asymptomatic group. When the analyses were done only on employed respondents, odds ratios indicated that minor depression appeared to be associated with an increased risk of disability days (this trend approached conventional levels of statistical significance). All of the preceding odds ratio analyses controlled for a number of potentially relevant variables, such as presence of chronic medical illnesses, social support, and demographic variables. It must be noted, however, that these analyses, like those of Wells et al. (1989), did not control for severity of medical illness.

Broadhead et al. (1990) concluded that "a significant proportion of persons with minor depression may have a disorder with similar functional impairments to major depressive disorder, or perhaps a milder form of that disorder, rather than a mild self-limiting adjustment reaction" (p. 16). They also noted that although the risk of disability was lower for those with minor depression than for those with major depression, "more disability days [are] attributable to minor depression due to its prevalence. Thus, the societal impact of minor depression may be greater than for major depression and dysthymia" (pp. 16–17).

Although statistical tests were not reported, large standard deviations in disability days of the group with minor depression (both total sample and employed persons only) are noteworthy (see Table 3 in Broadhead et al., 1990). The large standard deviations (e.g., 17.43) were associated with relatively small means (e.g., 4.45), suggesting that the group with minor depression was heterogeneous in terms of the relationship between depressed symptoms and functional impairment. One implication of this observation for a field trial on subthreshold minor depression is that it is important to identify patient characteristics that distinguish people who have functional impairment associated with their depressive symptoms from those who do not. Once again, since anxiety symptoms were "skipped," it is not possible to determine the percentage of this sample who also presented with anxious symptomatology, and therefore with MAD. However, the findings from Hiller et al. (1989), reviewed above, would suggest that this percentage would be very high.

To conclude this brief overview, the available evidence suggests that currently subdefinitional threshold cases of anxiety and depressive disorders are highly prevalent, particularly in primary care settings, and are associated with substantial impairment. However, methodological limitations of the previous studies in this area leave several important questions unanswered. Are the affective symptoms and impairment reported by these patients simply the consequence of medical conditions? What percentage of the cases of minor depression found in studies such as that of Broadhead et al. (1990) also presented with anxious symptomatology? What percentage of these supposedly subdefinitional threshold cases would actually have met diagnostic criteria for existing DSM-III-R categories if they had been assessed more thoroughly? In the remainder of this chapter, we describe the methods and procedures of the DSM-IV MAD field trial, which is designed to provide at least preliminary answers to these important questions. This field trial, with funding from the National Institute of Mental Health, is being carried out under our direction in collaboration with Michael Liebowitz, MD, as co-principal investigator.

THE DSM-IV MAD FIELD TRIAL

Overview

Although the ICD-10 includes a diagnostic category of MAD, no existing diagnostic system suggests diagnostic criteria for this category. Therefore, the two primary purposes of this field trial are (1) to identify criteria for the category of MAD through exploratory analyses; and (2) to investigate the reliability and validity of the proposed criteria. An empirical approach is being used to identify a reliable and valid set of diagnostic criteria for MAD. Toward this end, a combination of a criterion-oriented approach and the homogeneous-item approach to measurement (Nunnally, 1978) is being used. Although selecting items purely on the basis of correlations with a criterion is clearly inappropriate when constructing measures of theoretical constructs, a stronger case for adopting criterion-oriented approaches can be made in applied work. Nevertheless, we are following Nunnally's (1978) recommendation and are not ignoring correlations among items and considerations of internal consistency in selecting items for the proposed set of diagnostic criteria.

To accomplish the second goal, a common cross-validational strategy is being used to establish the reliability and validity of the proposed set of criteria. The sample is being split within each site (see below) into two groups. The data from the first group are to be used in an exploratory fashion to generate a set (or alternative sets) of diagnostic criteria; data from the second group are to be used to validate and estimate the reliability of the set(s) of criteria derived from the first group.

Design

Three sites, including two primary care sites (Baylor College of Medicine, New York State Psychiatric Institute) and one outpatient mental health site (the Phobia and Anxiety Disorders Clinic at the University at Albany, State University of New York), are participating in this field trial. All individuals referred to the three participating sites are screened on a brief self-administered questionnaire containing a 28-item scale of subjective distress and a 16-item impairment scale (see the "Measures" section, below). All individuals who exceed the cutoff on the subjective distress scale of this initial screening are evaluated and diagnosed, following DSM-III-R criteria. This evaluation consists of a comprehensive structured interview (the Anxiety Disorders Interview Schedule—Revised [ADIS-R]), and a battery of questionnaire measures of anxiety and depression and related constructs (affectivity or emotionality and cognitive style).

At least 150 patients are being fully evaluated at each of the three sites. All subjects who do not exceed the cutoff on the initial depression and anxiety screening comprise a comparison control group.

Half of the cross-validational sample cases at each site are being randomly assigned to have a second, independent diagnostic assessment, and several cases are being randomly audiotaped for each rater at each site. These audiotapes are to be rerated by raters at the other sites. These procedures should allow us to assess reliability both within and across sites.

Patient Recruitment, Selection, and Sample Size

Recruitment

The sites have been chosen in accordance with a model of deliberate sampling for heterogeneity with respect to the variables of specialty of care provider (primary care vs. outpatient mental health) and ethnicity. This strategy should enable us to examine differences as a function of these variables and to increase the external validity of the findings (Cook & Campbell, 1979).

Selection and Sample Size

Each site is being asked to administer a brief self-administered questionnaire (the 28-item General Health Questionnaire [GHQ]; Goldberg & Hillier, 1979) to all adult, English-speaking patients capable of completing self-administered questionnaires. A minimum of 150 subjects at each site are to be fully assessed after exceeding the cutoff on this screening, to identify those patients at elevated risk of presenting with subdefinitional MAD, minor depression, or adjustment disorders with anxious and/or depressed mood. In addition, we are collecting data regarding social and occupational or school functioning from all subjects at each site, regardless of whether or not they exceed the cutoff on the brief screening.

Consistent with the conservative approach underlying this field trial and with the procedures of Broadhead et al. (1990), we are excluding those subjects whose symptoms on the screening can be explained by an emergent major medical illness, medication, or drug or alcohol use. Thus, subjects who report an onset of depressive or anxious symptoms within 6 months of the onset of diagnosis of a major medical illness are being excluded. Since the majority of the patients seen at the primary care settings are seen for routine monitoring or treatment maintenance of a stable, chronic illness, we do not anticipate that these conservative exclusion criteria should interfere with our ability to generate the desired sample sizes. For example, at one of the primary care clinics affiliated with the New York State Psychiatric Institute, 50% of the patients are seen for routine maintenance or monitoring of hypertension, and another 25% are seen for routine maintenance or monitoring of diabetes.

On the basis of previous research (Goldberg & Hillier, 1979; Von Korff et al., 1987; Wells et al., 1989), we estimate that 20–40% of the patients at the primary care sites will exceed the screening cutoff. Thus, we estimate that the brief screen will be administered to between 375 and 750 patients at each primary care site, to generate the desired minimum number of subjects receiving the full assessment battery at each site. We anticipate that the majority of subjects at the Albany site will exceed the screening cutoff; however, relevant data will be available from a sample of "normal" controls who are being recruited for another ongoing research project at the Albany clinic. Aggregated across each of the sites, we therefore expect minimum samples of 450 patients who will exceed the screening cutoff, and between 700 and 1,825 individuals who will receive the screening but not exceed the screening cutoff.

Measures

The most important of the measures included in the field trial are the following:

General Health Questionnaire

The 28-item version of the GHQ (Goldberg & Hillier, 1979) is a self-report instrument designed to identify persons likely to have a psychiatric disorder characterized by subjective distress. Versions of the GHQ have been used widely in studies of primary care patients (e.g., Goldberg & Hillier, 1979; Von Korff et al., 1987). Although factor analyses indicate that the GHQ may be broken into four subscales, the four subscales are by no means independent of each other, and there is strong evidence of one general factor that runs through the items (Goldberg & Hillier, 1979). In addition, total scores on the GHQ have been found to be positively related to the likelihood of a clinical diagnosis of a psychiatric disorder from a structured interview (Goldberg & Hillier, 1979). Following the recommendations of Goldberg and Hillier (1979), we are scoring items on a dichotomous basis (0 or 1), and we are using a total score of 5 or greater as the cutting point for identifying the sample of high-risk individuals to receive further assessment (see also Von Korff et al., 1987, for a replication of the usefulness of this cutting score).

Rand Impairment Measure

The Rand Impairment Measure (Stewart, Hays, & Ware, 1988; Wells et al., 1989) is a self-report instrument eliciting information on six domains of functioning: "physical," "role (work or school)," "social," "bed days," "well-being," and "free of pain." All measures except days in bed are scored from 0 to 100, with 100 representing perfect health on that construct. The "bed days" measure is the number of days spent in bed in the past 30 days. A more detailed description of these measures is available in Stewart et al. (1988).

Anxiety Disorders Interview Schedule—Revised

The ADIS-R (Di Nardo & Barlow, 1988) is being used at all sites to determine whether patients meet the current DSM-III-R diagnostic criteria for a depressive disorder or an anxiety disorder. The same diagnostic procedure is being used across sites to ensure similar sample selection with respect to diagnostic status. Psychometric studies based on two independent diagnostic interviews indicate that adequate reliabilities can be obtained for the DSM-III-R depressive disorders and anxiety disorders (Barlow, 1988).

Versions of the Hamilton Rating Scale (HARS) and the Hamilton Rating Scale for Depression (HRSD) are being revised for this field trial. The ADIS-R includes the HARS and HRSD as well as the revised HARS and HRSD (Riskind, Beck, Brown, & Steer, 1987; see also Chapter 8), which were developed to reduce the amount of overlap between the HARS and the HRSD and thereby to distinguish more clearly between anxiety and depression. The additional revisions for this field trial consist of incorporating items derived from RDC minor depression criteria and DSM-III-R anxiety disorders criteria from the ADIS-R that do not overlap with current Hamilton Rating Scale items.

Procedure

Eligible patients who agree to participate are scheduled for an assessment session. The interviewer describes the procedures involved in the study and asks each patient to read (and, if willing to participate, to sign) an informed consent statement. The interviewer then administers the ADIS-

R. Patients who are to be re-evaluated to examine interrater reliability are scheduled for a second ADIS-R 1 one week later. After patients have completed the assessment study, they are referred promptly for appropriate treatment of their presenting problem.

Data Analyses

Establishing Diagnostic Criteria

To ensure that the proposed category of MAD does not include individuals experiencing normal anxious and depressed affect, we will correlate each of the potential criteria with impairment scores and will select only those items that effectively discriminate impaired from unimpaired individuals. Thus, the first step in the data analyses will be geared to establishing a useful cutoff point for separating individuals into impaired and unimpaired groups. To accomplish this goal, the initial analyses will involve examining the univariate distribution of a total impairment index (summed across all six domains of functioning) for evidence that the observed distribution results from the sampling of two (or more) distinct populations.

Evidence consistent with the existence of distinct populations will result if what Grove and Andreasen (1989) have called "bitangentiality" is observed. Bitangentiality consists of requiring that there be bimodality, or that there be two distinct tangents to the distribution curve on one side of the mode of a unimodal distribution (see Figure 7.1). In other words, bitangentiality occurs when there is more than one "hump" in a distribution. If observed, bitangentiality will identify what Kendell (1975) has called "a point of rarity" and will indicate that the impairment scores are indeed coming from separate populations—a normal population and a disordered population (or populations). This point of rarity can then be used as a cutting score on the impairment distribution that separates the two populations with the minimal amount of overlap that is possible (see below for more details).

One potential problem with the search for bitangentiality among the observed impairment scores is that such "lumpy" distributions (i.e., containing more than one hump) may be obtained at the observed level even when the distribution of the underlying latent trait is not "lumpy." Grayson (1987) has demonstrated that this will occur if the items tapping the latent trait cluster in their endorsement rates at a similar point of the latent distribution. Individuals falling below this point will form one hump at the low end of the observed scale, whereas individuals above this point will form a distinct hump at the high end of the observed scale. To rule out this possibility, a statistical model derived from item response theory (Lord & Novick, 1968; Rasch, 1969; Wright, 1977) will be used to

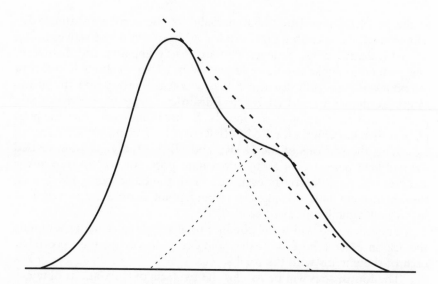

FIGURE 7.1. A distribution showing bitangentiality. From Grove, W., & Andreason, N. (1989). Quantitative and qualitative distinctions between psychiatric disorders. In L. N. Robins & J. E. Barrett (Eds.), *The validity of psychiatric diagnosis*. New York: Raven Press. Copyright 1989 by Raven Press, Ltd. Reprinted by permission.

estimate the distribution of the latent impairment scores from the observed impairment scores, and the estimated latent distribution will be examined for bitangentiality.

If the latent impairment distribution demonstrates bitangentiality, the first hump may be interpreted as belonging to a "normal" population, and the second may be interpreted as belonging to a "disordered" population. Thus, the least frequently observed impairment value between the first two humps represents a useful cutting point, since the probability that an individual comes from the normal population is greater than the probability that he or she comes from the disordered population up to that point, and vice versa beyond that point.

The approach described above will obviously have to be modified if the distribution of latent impairment scores does not display bitangentiality. Unitangentiality, if observed, will be consistent with a continuity model of psychopathology, in which "pathological" traits and characteristics are continuously distributed throughout the population.[1] One practical solution

---

[1] As noted by Grove and Andreasen (1989), unitangentiality may still be formally compatible with a discontinuity model, since two separate population distributions that are separated only modestly may together comprise a unitangential mixed sample distribution.

to the problems posed by unitangentiality of the latent impairment distribution will be to choose a more or less arbitrary but conservative cutting point to identify those patients who are clearly impaired and distressed. One method to implement this solution will be to plot the latent impairment distributions separately for the Albany "normal" group and the group meeting criteria for DSM-III-R Axis I disorders, and to choose the cutting point so that all individuals scoring above that point come from the population meeting criteria for DSM-III-R Axis I disorders.

With the versions of the HARS and HRSD that have been revised for this field trial serving as an initial item pool, the second step in the analyses will be to correlate each item with the dichotomized scores on the impairment index (using the cutting point derived from step 1 to dichotomize the impairment scores).

The third step will be to obtain a total symptom score by summing the responses to each of the anxiety and depression items, and to correlate each of these items with the total score.

The fourth step will be to plot the two sets of correlations obtained from steps 2 and 3, and to select those items that correlate most highly with both the criterion and with total scores.

The final step will be to arrive at a decision rule that relates the clinical features to the diagnostic category. To do so, the performance of several alternative decision rules (e.g., presence of at least two symptoms vs. at least three symptoms, etc.) and duration criteria (1 week vs. 2 weeks, etc.) in terms of their correlations with the dichotomized impairment scores will be compared to select the rule with the greatest specificity and sensitivity.

Reliability

To examine the internal consistency of the proposed criteria, we will examine the item–total correlations, Cronbach's (1951) coefficient alpha, and an estimate of homogeneity based on principal-components analysis (Zinbarg & Revelle, 1991).

To examine interrater reliability, one-half of the cases from the cross-validational sample at each site will be randomly assigned to have a second, independent diagnostic assessment within 1 week of the first diagnostic assessment. The interrater reliability will be assessed separately for diagnoses made in the primary care sites by diagnosticians who are experienced in the assessment of DSM-III-R mood, anxiety, and adjustment disorders, and by diagnosticians who are trained to administer the interviews but have less prior experience in assessing anxious and depressed patients with the DSM-III-R system.

Validity

Functional impairment, as assessed by the method used in the Rand Outcome Study (Stewart et al., 1988; Wells et al., 1989), will be the primary external validation criterion in the cross-validational sample. The primary analysis of the data on functional impairment will examine the relationship between group status (current DSM-III-R Axis I disorder, current MAD, no current DSM-III-R Axis I or MAD) and a total impairment index (summing across the six domains of functioning), with the presence and/or severity of recent life stressors and medical conditions partialed or covaried out.

The use of a structured diagnostic interview to make diagnoses will enable us to examine the discriminant validity of the proposed category and its diagnostic criteria. That is, we will be able to assess the possibility that primary care patients described in prior studies as potentially having subclinical anxiety and depression or minor depression meet diagnostic criteria for existing DSM-III-R categories.

The relationship between group status (DSM-III-R major depressive episode, DSM-III-R anxiety disorders, MAD, DSM-III-R adjustment disorder with depressed and/or anxious mood, and no disorder) and extent (and, if possible, type) of family history of psychopathology will also be examined. Evidence for the construct validity of the MAD category, if found, will consist of the MAD group's being more similar to the groups with DSM-III-R major depressive episode and anxiety disorders than to the groups with adjustment disorder and no disorder in their family history.

Finally, examination of the duration and age at onset should provide preliminary evidence regarding the distinction between the proposed MAD category and DSM-III-R Axis II conditions. Thus, if the MAD group does not differ substantially from the DSM-III-R Axis I groups on either of these variables, and their typical age of onset is not in early adulthood, then it should appear that the category under investigation can be distinguished from Axis II conditions (pending further study).

Prevalence

Prevalence estimates for the primary care sites will be derived in three ways: (1) based on all patients who are evaluated at each site, (2) based on all patients who complete the initial screening, and (3) based only on those who exceed the initial screening cutoff. Prevalence estimates for the outpatient mental health clinic site will be based on all patients who are evaluated at the clinic. Prevalence differences as a function of gender, ethnicity, and type of site (primary care vs. outpatient mental health clinic) will be analyzed by hierarchical multiple regression, following procedures recommended by Cohen and Cohen (1983).

CONCLUSIONS

A great deal of evidence suggests that there may be many patients with symptoms of anxiety and/or depression and substantial impairment that do not meet current definitional thresholds for Axis I anxiety or mood disorders. However, several important questions regarding these cases need to be answered before we revise the existing diagnostic nomenclature to include them. Are the depressive and/or anxious features and impairment experienced by these individuals simply consequences of medical conditions? If these cases are carefully assessed by mental health professionals using structured diagnostic interviews, will the majority of them meet diagnostic criteria for existing DSM-III-R Axis I anxiety or mood disorders?

From the outset of our investigation, we caution that a search for MAD and/or minor depression raises some of the most basic and challenging questions in the field of psychopathology. What is a useful diagnostic category? How can we determine whether a hypothesized diagnostic category exists in nature? In other words, how can we ensure that we are carving nature at its joints? For that matter, does nature have "joints"? That is, can categorical and dimensional or continuity models of psychopathology be distinguished? We do not have all the answers to these complex questions, nor are we convinced that "the" answer to any of these questions exists. However, we suggest that at a methodological level, recent advances in psychometric theory and techniques may provide invaluable tools in our efforts to arrive at a useful and valid nosology. In this chapter, we have illustrated how the concept of bitangentiality and latent trait models can be used to discover a "point of rarity," if it exists, with respect to the important external criterion of functional impairment. Applications of these psychometric methods and principles to psychodiagnosis should enhance our understanding of the nature of what currently appears to be a subdefinitional subset of the anxiety and depressive disorders.

REFERENCES

American Psychiatric Association. (1987). *Diagnostic and statistical manual of mental disorders* (3rd ed., rev.). Washington, DC: Author.

Barlow, D. H. (1988). *Anxiety and its disorders: The nature and treatment of anxiety and panic*. New York: Guilford Press.

Barrett, J. E., Barrett, J. A., Oxman, T. E., & Gerber, P. D. (1988). The prevalence of psychiatric disorders in a primary care practice. *Archives of General Psychiatry*, *45*, 1100–1106.

Broadhead, W. E., Blazer, D., George, L., & Kit Tse, C. (1990). Depression, disability days, and days lost from work in a prospective epidemiologic survey. *Journal of American Medical Association*, *264*, 2524–2528.

Clark, D. A., & Watson, D. (1990). *Psychometric issues relevant to a potential DSM-IV category of mixed anxiety–depression.* Unpublished manuscript, DSM-IV Subgroup on Generalized Anxiety Disorder and Mixed Anxiety–Depression.

Cohen, J., & Cohen, P. (1983). *Applied multiple regression/correlation analysis for the behavioral sciences.* Hillsdale, NJ: Erlbaum.

Cook, T. D., & Campbell, D. T. (1979). *Quasi-experimentation: Design and analysis issues for field settings.* Boston: Houghton Mifflin.

Cronbach, L. (1951). Coefficient alpha and the internal structure of tests. *Psychometrika*, *16*, 297–334.

Di Nardo, P. A., & Barlow, D. H. (1988). *Anxiety Disorders Interview Schedule—Revised (ADIS-R).* Albany: Center for Stress and Anxiety Disorders, University at Albany, State University of New York.

Dohrenwend, B., Shrout, P. E., Egri, G., & Mendelsohn, F. S. (1980). Nonspecific psychological distress and other dimensions of psychopathology: Measures for use in the general population. *Archives of General Psychiatry*, *37*, 1229–1236.

Eaton, W. W., McCutcheon, A., Dryman, & Sorenson, A. (in press). Latent-class analysis: Anxiety and depression sociological methods and research.

Goldberg, D., & Hillier, V. C. (1979). A scaled version of the General Health Questionnaire. *Psychological Medicine*, *9*, 139–145.

Grayson, D. A. (1987). Can categorical and dimensional views of psychiatric illness be distinguished? *British Journal of Psychiatry*, *151*, 355–361.

Grove, W., & Andreasen, N. (1989). Quantitative and qualitative distinctions between psychiatric disorders. In L. N. Robins & J. E. Barrett (Eds.), *The validity of psychiatric diagnosis.* New York: Raven Press.

Hiller, W., Zaudig, M., & Bose, M. (1989). The overlap between depression and anxiety on different levels of psychopathology. *Journal of Affective Disorders*, *16*, 223–231.

Katon, W., & Roy-Byrne, P. (1989). *Mixed anxiety and depression.* Unpublished manuscript, DSM-IV Subgroup on Generalized Anxiety Disorder and Mixed Anxiety–Depression.

Kendell, R. E. (1975). *The role of diagnosis in psychiatry.* Oxford: Blackwell Scientific.

Klerman, G. L. (1989). Depressive disorders: Further evidence for increased medical morbidity and impairment of social functioning. *Archives of General Psychiatry*, *46*, 856–858.

Lord, F., & Novick, M. (1968). *Statistical theories of mental test scores.* Reading, MA: Addison-Wesley.

Nunnally, J. (1978). *Psychometric theory* (2nd ed.). New York: McGraw-Hill.

Rasch, G. (1960). *Probabilistic models for some intelligence and attainment tests.* Copenhagen: Danmarks Paedogogisheh Institut.

Riskind, J. H., Beck, A. T., Brown, G., & Steer, R. A. (1987). Taking the measure of anxiety and depression: Validity of the reconstructed Hamilton Rating Scales. *Journal of Nervous and Mental Disease, 175,* 474–479.

Stewart, A., Hays, R., & Ware, J. (1988). The MOS short-form General Health Survey. *Medical Care, 26,* 724–735.

Tellegen, A. (1985). Structures of mood and personality and their relevance to assessing anxiety, with an emphasis on self-report. In A. H. Tuma & J. D. Maser (Eds.), *Anxiety and the anxiety disorders.* Hillsdale, NJ: Erlbaum.

Von Korff, M., Shapiro, S., Burke, J., Teitlebaum, M., Skinner, E., German, P., Turner, R., Klein, L., & Burns, B. (1987). Anxiety and depression in a primary care clinic: Comparison of Diagnostic Interview Schedule, General Health Questionnaire and Practitioner Assessments. *Archives of General Psychiatry, 44,* 152–156.

Wells, K., Stewart, A., Hays, R., Burnam, A., Rogers, W., Daniels, M., Berry, S., Greenfield, S., & Ware, J. (1989). The functioning and well-being of depressed patients. *Journal of the American Medical Association, 262,* 914–919.

Wright, B. (1977). Solving measurement problems with the Rosch model. *Journal of Educational Measurement, 14,* 97–116.

Zinbarg, R. E., & Revelle, W. (1991). *The first factor saturation index (FFS) and the internal structure of tests.* Manuscript in preparation.

8

The Relation of Generalized Anxiety Disorder to Depression in General and Dysthymic Disorder in Particular

JOHN H. RISKIND
ROGER MOORE
BILL HARMAN
George Mason University

ANN A. HOHMANN
National Institute of Mental Health

AARON T. BECK
BONNIE STEWART
University of Pennsylvania School of Medicine

The field of psychopathology has witnessed long debate about the relation of anxiety to depression. The same debate influences the forthcoming construction of the DSM-IV category of generalized anxiety disorder (GAD). One chief question about GAD has been whether signs and symptoms permit the practicing clinician to discriminate this anxiety disorder from depression in general, and from dysthymic disorder (DD) in particular.*

* The name of this disorder became simply "dysthymia" with the publication of the revised third edition of the *Diagnostic and Statistical Manual of Mental Disorders* (DSM-III-R) in 1987. However, we are abbreviating it as "DD" in this chapter—not only for the sake of brevity, but because the data sets to be described later employed both DSM-III ("dysthymic disorder") and DSM-III-R ("dysthymia") criteria.

This chapter is based upon an unpublished paper for the DSM-IV Subgroup on Generalized Anxiety Disorder and Mixed Anxiety–Depression.

153

To be sure, DD is a particularly challenging comparison for GAD, because it too is a chronic form of affective disturbance. Nonetheless, identifying signs and symptoms that facilitate the differential diagnosis of GAD from DD would bolster the practical utility of the category of GAD.

This chapter summarizes the results of a literature review and preliminary analysis of two data sets on this clinical question. First, we briefly review the relation of GAD to depression in general, then devote the remainder of the chapter to examining its specific relation to DD.

RELATION OF GAD TO DEPRESSION IN GENERAL

Previous research has found considerable evidence that GAD is related to depression. Indeed, patients with GAD often present with depression (Hoehn-Saric & McLeod, 1985; Barlow, Di Nardo, Vermilyea, Vermilyea, & Blanchard, 1986). In fact, studies by the Newcastle group in Great Britain, prior to the publication of DSM-III, found that depressive symptoms appeared in as many as 65% of patients with "anxiety neurosis" (Roth, Gurney, Garside, & Kerr, 1972). Moreover, several studies have found "secondary" depression in anxious patients (Clancy, Noyes, Hoenk, & Slymen, 1979; Dealy, Ishiiki, Avery, Wilson, & Dunner, 1981; Winokur, 1988). Furthermore, a recent study by Barlow's Albany group, using DSM-III criteria, found comorbidity with formal depression disorders, including major depression (MD) and DD, in 17% of the diagnosed cases of GAD (Barlow, Di Nardo, et al., 1986).

Of course, overlap does not necessarily indicate that disorders are interchangeable. A few years ago, it was argued that GAD and MD are related so closely that they cannot be meaningfully discriminated from each other (Breier, Charney, & Heninger, 1985). Nonetheless, several studies suggested that significant differences discriminate the symptoms of GAD and MD (Riskind, Beck, Brown, & Steer, 1987; Beck, Brown, Steer, Eidelson, Riskind, 1987).

REASONS FOR COMPARING GAD AND DD

As disorders, GAD and DD are interesting because they may be harder to discriminate than GAD and MD: Both are low-grade, cross-situational forms of affective disturbances. Both show chronicity, so that patients with GAD as well as those with DD have been anxious for a large part of their lives (Barlow, Blanchard, Vermilyea, Vermilyea, & Di Nardo, 1986; Rapee, 1990). Moreover, the unique diagnostic status of both disorders has been doubted, because both are potential prodromes for disorders such as MD or panic (see Chapter 1). Finally, it has been similarly questioned whether either GAD (Breier et al., 1985) or DD is really distinct from MD (Weissman, Leaf, Bruce, & Florio, 1988). Therefore, GAD and DD seem to share many features.

Several studies suggest the possible symptom overlap. For example, anxiety symptoms are a part of the profile in at least one subgroup of patients with DD (Parker, Blignault, & Manicavasagar, 1988; Klein, Taylor, Dickstein, & Harding, 1988), much as the symptoms are also a part of the profile in a subgroup of patients with MD (Fawcett & Kravitz, 1983; Garvey, Cook, & Noyes, 1989). Indeed, Di Nardo and Barlow (1990) have found that an additional GAD diagnosis occurs in about 45% of the cases of MD and 33% of the cases of DD. Moreover, a community study found that more than 75% of individuals with DD had other disorders, particularly MD and anxiety disorders (Weissman et al., 1988). The same overlap has been observed in GAD. Thus, depressive symptoms are often an important part of the profile in at least one subgroup of GADs (Hoehn-Saric & McLeod, 1985; Barlow, Di Nardo, et al., 1986).

The previous studies raise important questions about the symptom overlap between GAD and DD, yet stop too short to permit a direct evaluation. The evaluation of that overlap is the main purpose of the remainder of this chapter.

OVERVIEW OF STUDY METHODOLOGY

We examined the question of whether GAD and DD can be discriminated by means of their presenting symptoms in two ways. The first approach involved a systematic literature search for published studies comparing GAD and DD. The second method consisted of a search for unpublished data sets that could shed light on the boundary between the disorders.

LITERATURE SEARCH OF PUBLISHED STUDIES

The computer search was done with Medline and PsycLit (in the psychiatric and psychological literature, respectively), using terms such as "generalized anxiety," "dysthymia/dysthymic disorder," "anxiety and depression," "anxiety neurosis," and "GAD," and covering the years from 1980 to the present. It focused on key English-language journal articles involving human subjects; the journals included the *Journal of Affective Disorders*, *Archives of General Psychiatry*, *Journal of Abnormal Psychology*, *American Journal of Psychiatry*,

British Journal of Psychiatry, Journal of Anxiety Disorders, and others. Shelf copies were reviewed "manually" for the past 8 years, or until their first issues. Moreover, additional sources were explored by reviewing bibliographic references in recent articles and review papers, and contacting known investigators and groups for pertinent manuscripts.

The review found several published articles including DSM-III or DSM-III-R categories for both GAD and DD, but none of the articles compared signs and symptoms of the disorders. Relevant data had not been collected in some studies. Studies of chronic depression and chronic anxiety by the Newcastle group (e.g., Roth et al., 1972; Roth, Mountjoy, & Caetano, 1982), and others, were disqualified because they did not apply DSM-III or DSM-III-R criteria.

Search for Unpublished Data Sets

Our search for unpublished data, in which we contacted known investigators, produced two relevant data sets. One was from the Center for Cognitive Therapy in Philadelphia (CCT; Beck's group). The other data set was from the Center for Stress and Anxiety Disorders in Albany (CSAD; Barlow's group). Both data sets allowed us to compare whether presenting symptoms discriminate GAD and DD.

Philadelphia Data Set

Sample. The CCT sample, from Philadelphia, included data from 518 clinic outpatients. All outpatients were diagnosed with either DSM-III or DSM-III-R criteria, using the Structured Clinical Interview for DSM-III/DSM-III-R (SCID) of Spitzer and Williams (Spitzer & Williams, 1983; Spitzer, Williams, & Gibbon, 1987). If DSM-III criteria were used, comorbid diagnoses were allowed when the disorders were independent. Therefore, the DSM-III decision rules precluding certain comorbid diagnoses were suspended (see Spitzer & Williams, 1985; Barlow, Di Nardo, et al., 1986). The patients included in the data set had one or more of the following diagnoses: GAD, DD, panic disorder, MD.

The principal analyses focused only on those patients who had a primary diagnosis (DSM-III or DSM-III-R) of either "pure" GAD ($n =$ 26) or pure DD ($n = 31$) alone. Consequently, these patients had no additional Axis I diagnoses.

Subsidiary analyses were also carried out on two larger and "impure" groups: patients who had any diagnosis—primary, secondary, or tertiary—of either "mixed" GAD ($n = 156$) or "mixed" DD ($n = 104$). To illustrate, any patient with a secondary diagnosis of GAD was included in the GAD group, even if the patient's primary diagnosis was MD. Nevertheless, these mixed groups were mutually exclusive: No patients with GAD had a diagnosis of DD, or vice versa. The measures included revised versions (Riskind et al., 1987) of the Hamilton Anxiety Rating Scale (Hamilton, 1959) and the Hamilton Rating Scale for Depression (Hamilton, 1960); the Beck Anxiety Inventory (Beck, Epstein, Brown, & Steer, 1988); the Beck Depression Inventory (BDI; Beck, Ward, Mendelson, Mock, & Erbaugh, 1961); the Hopelessness Scale (Beck, Weissman, Lester, & Trexler, 1974); the Scale for Suicide Ideation (Beck, Kovacs, & Weissman, 1979); the Cognitions Checklist Anxiety and Depression subscales (Beck et al., 1987); the Rosenbaum Self-Control Schedule (Rosenbaum, 1980); the Dysfunctional Attitude Scale (Weissman & Beck, 1978); and the Clarke Institute of Psychiatry version of the Wechsler Adult Intelligence Scale (WAIS) Vocabulary subtest (Patich & Crawford).

The analyses focused on the nondemographic information, a large proportion of the demographic data being missing. The GAD subjects tended to be slightly less well educated than the DD subjects, and analyses likewise revealed that they had significantly lower scores (means = 30.23 vs. 33.37) on the Clarke WAIS Vocabulary subtest ($p < .03$). Thus, those data provided possible hints of differences between the GAD and DD subjects.

Results.

1. *"Pure" GAD and DD groups.* Within this CCT sample, the "pure" cases of GAD and DD could be discriminated by global presenting symptoms. As would be expected from the criteria contained in the DSM-III or DSM-III-R, the GAD subjects had generally higher anxiety symptoms than did the DD subjects, on both the Beck Anxiety Inventory (means = 16.04 vs. 11.50) and the revised Hamilton Anxiety Rating Scale (means = 14.77 vs. 7.65) (both p's < .0003). Conversely, the DD subjects had generally higher depression symptoms than did the GAD subjects, on both the BDI (means = 19.55 vs. 12.04) and the revised Hamilton Rating Scale for Depression (means = 11.23 vs. 6.65) (both p's < .0001). Therefore, the "pure" groups could be discriminated by anxiety and depression.

Different profiles of the symptoms were also found on the items of the two Hamilton scales. First, as expected (see Table 8.1), the GAD group showed significantly higher autonomic and respiratory symptoms, and agitation and motor tension, than did the DD group. Nonetheless, not all the differences upheld the expectations for GAD. Most obviously, the GAD subjects failed to show higher symptoms of apprehensive fears and gastrointestinal complaints than did the DD subjects.

Second, and also as expected, the DD subjects exhibited higher depression symptoms of depressed mood, suicidal ideation, guilt, and work

TABLE 8.1. Individual Symptoms for the Pure GAD and DD Groups in Philadelphia

	DD group mean ($n = 31$)	GAD group mean ($n = 26$)	Probability from t test
Hamilton Anxiety items			
1. Anxious mood	1.45	1.79	.10
2. Tension	1.23	1.69	.04
3. Fears	0.58	0.92	.11
4. Insomnia	0.68	1.04	.12
5. Intellectual	0.83	1.08	.26
6. Depressed mood	1.74	0.81	.0001
7. Somatic: muscular	0.42	0.96	.005
8. Somatic: sensory	0.10	0.60	.001
9. Cardiovascular	0.26	1.08	.0001
10. Respiratory	0.13	0.73	.0027
11. Gastrointestinal	0.58	0.85	.22
12. Genitourinary	0.23	0.58	.05
13. Autonomic	0.26	0.92	.0003
14. Behavior at interview	0.58	1.28	.0005
Hamilton Depression items			
1. Depressed mood	1.90	0.67	.0001
2. Feelings of guilt	1.23	0.84	.03
3. Suicide	0.42	0.04	.02
4. Insomnia: early	0.16	0.28	.34
5. Insomnia: middle	0.52	0.28	.16
6. Insomnia: late	0.19	0.36	.24
7. Work and activities	1.42	0.64	.0002
8. Retardation	0.32	0.16	.27
9. Agitation	0.19	0.52	.02
10. Anxiety: psychic	0.90	1.48	.008
11. Anxiety: somatic	0.48	1.28	.0002
12. Somatic: gastrointestinal	0.10	0.24	.20
13. Somatic: general	0.26	0.64	.02
14. Genital	0.29	0.32	.83
15. Hypochondriasis	0.19	0.48	.12
16. Loss of weight	0.03	0.08	.55
17. Insight	0.13	0.00	—
18. Diurnal variation (A.M.)	0.52	0.19	.02
19. Diurnal variation (P.M.)	0.34	0.13	.09
20. Depersonalization	0.06	0.32	.08
21. Paranoid	0.32	0.12	.21
22. Obsessive–compulsive	0.26	0.28	.86
23. Helplessness	1.03	1.04	.97
24. Hopelessness	1.48	0.72	.002
25. Worthlessness	1.50	0.76	.001

impairment than did the GAD subjects. The DD group also showed higher hopelessness and worthlessness on the Hamilton scale items.

For the full-fledged measures of depressive cognitions, the DD group had higher scores than the GAD group on both the Cognitions Checklist Depression subscale (means = 25.97 vs. 12.20), and the Hopelessness Scale (means = 11.58 vs. 6.08) (both *p*'s < .0001). Such outcomes could certainly have been predicted from cognitive models of affective disorders (e.g., Beck et al., 1987). But the outcomes for the full-fledged measures of anxiety cognitions were inconsistent with such models: Repeating the null outcomes with the "fearful apprehension" items on the Hamilton Anxiety Rating Scale, the GAD subjects failed to have higher scores than the DD subjects on the Cognitions Checklist Anxiety subscale (means = 15.52 vs. 15.17) (n.s.). Therefore, anxious cognitions were less discriminating than depressive cognitions at separating the two disorders.

Moreover, the DD group also had a lower mean score on the Rosenbaum Self-Control Schedule (−3.11) than the GAD group (6.23) (*p* < .04), and a higher mean score on the Scale for Suicide Ideation—Worst Rating (6.53) than the GAD group (1.44) (*p* < .0001). These differences are consistent with the hopelessness findings described above. Moreover, the mean score of the DD group (370.86) was slightly higher than that of the GAD group (327.88) on the Dysfunctional Attitudes Scale (*p* < .09). Therefore, several other cognitive measures also seemed to discriminate the DD subjects from the GAD subjects.

Further analyses confirmed that the presenting symptoms could predict the DSM diagnostic classifications received by the pure groups. In fact, a discriminant function analysis on the revised scores of Riskind et al. (1987) for the two Hamilton scales revealed that general anxiety and depression symptoms correctly classified 92.3% of the cases with a GAD diagnosis, and 83.9% of those with a DD diagnosis.

A few core symptoms of GAD were selected to explore whether they contributed to the prediction of the diagnostic classifications. These included psychic anxiety (Hamilton Depression item 10), autonomic symptoms (Hamilton Anxiety item 13), and cardiovascular symptoms (Hamilton Anxiety Item 9). When a hierarchical (or weighted) logistic model was applied, it revealed that each symptom contributed to discriminating the pure cases of GAD and DD (the *p*'s were .09, .024, and .017, respectively), with a model χ^2 (3) = 21.91, *p* < .05.

Next, a discriminant-function analysis was done, and it showed both the sensitivity and specificity of this logistic model in predicting a diagnosis of pure GAD or DD. In fact, the symptoms correctly classified the majority of the pure cases of GAD (75%) and DD (83.9%) in their categories.

2. *"Mixed" or comorbid groups*. With regard to outcomes, the "mixed" groups paralleled the "pure" groups, with three exceptions. First, the mixed GAD and DD subjects failed to differ on the BDI (means = 20.83 for the GAD group vs. 21.10 for the DD group) (n.s.), although they did differ significantly on the revised Hamilton Rating Scale for Depression (means = 10.43 for the GAD group vs. 12.74 for the DD group) ($p <$ .0001). Second, the outcomes for several classic symptoms of depression attained significance, but were directly opposite to expectation: Namely, the mixed GAD subjects reported greater problems both with "weight loss" (means = 0.33 for the GAD group vs. 0.10 for the DD group) ($p <$ .001) and with "late insomnia" (means = 0.51 for the GAD group vs. 0.34 for the DD group) ($p < $ .04) than did the mixed DD subjects on the Hamilton Rating Scale for Depression. Third and last, the outcomes for the measures of anxious cognition with the mixed groups now supported the cognitive models: The mixed GAD subjects had higher mean scores than did the mixed DD subjects on both the Cognitions Checklist Anxiety subscale (19.89 for the GAD group vs. 15.33 for the DD group) ($p <$ .0004), and the Hamilton Anxiety items 1 and 3) for apprehensive fears (1.92 for the GAD group vs. 1.56 for the DD group on item 1, and 0.97 for the GAD group vs. 0.54 for the DD group on item 3) (both p's $<$ .003).

In short, although no such outcome was found for the pure groups, the mixed GAD subjects displayed more anxious cognitions than the mixed DD subjects, as well as higher scores for certain depressive symptoms (e.g., weight loss, insomnia).

Possible Limitations of the Philadelphia Data. The results so far have several potential limitations that must be noted. First, only 26 "pure" cases of GAD, and 31 of DD, were obtained at the Philadelphia site; larger pure groups are obviously needed in the future. Second, females with DD usually predominate in the past literature; however, there was a puzzling preponderance here of males with DD (approximately 60%), which raises doubts about the representativeness of the cases. Third, the pure GAD sample combined cases that were diagnosed by both versions of DSM-III, which could introduce a confound: That is, GAD is defined as a *chronic* or continuous disorder (for 6 months) in DSM-III-R, but as a short-term disorder (for 1 month) in DSM-III.

Nevertheless, existing evidence weakens the possibility that differential chronicity confounds the results. Indeed, Sanderson and Barlow (1990) showed that 22 of 23 GAD cases diagnosed by DSM-III criteria in their clinic also met the DSM-III-R criteria. Therefore, within a clinical setting, it seems that nearly all cases of GAD that meet DSM-III criteria fulfill DSM-III-R criteria.

Albany Data Set

Sample. This chapter's second data set was provided by the Albany CSAD, as analyzed by Benshoof, Moras, Di Nardo, and Barlow (1990). Nearly all of their sample (*n* = 15 in each group) of mixed GAD and mixed DD subjects had comorbid disorders. The Albany data set also included other disorders (e.g., panic groups with and without agoraphobia), but these are not of interest in the present chapter.

All patients in the Albany sample were diagnosed with the Anxiety Disorders Interview Schedule—Revised (ADIS-R; Di Nardo & Barlow, 1988), and depressed patients also received the Schedule for Affective Disorders and Schizophrenia (Endicott & Spitzer, 1978). Analyses by Benshoof et al. were available for the items from the reconstructed Hamilton scales (Riskind et al., 1987), the BDI (Beck et al., 1961), and other scales (see Benshoof et al., 1990, for details).

The only significant demographic difference between the DSM-III-R categories of interest was for number of dependents living on the family income: Namely, the GAD subjects reported fewer dependents (mean = 1.7) living on the family income than did the DD subjects (mean = 3.4) ($p < .05$). No other demographic variables discriminated GAD and DD subjects. In fact, Benshoof et al. found no differences in gender, age, income level, number of children, years married, or educational level.

Results. In comparison to the outcomes of the Philadelphia CCT sample, Benshoof et al. (1990) found few differences in the Albany sample between the GAD and DD subjects. They found no differences in anxiety and depression on the Hamilton scales, the BDI, or other relevant measures. Nevertheless, the direction and magnitude of the differences on the BDI were consistent with those that found in the Philadelphia sample (means = 20.43 for the DD group vs. 14.33 for the GAD group). Thus Benshoof et al. might have found differences on the BDI if their sample sizes had been larger; as noted above, there were only 15 subjects in each group.

Benshoof et al. did not report the overall means for the revised Hamilton scoring system, but they did find a few significant differences in specific symptoms. Indeed, most symptoms failed to discriminate the groups. Nevertheless, higher respiratory symptoms (means = 1.23 vs. 0.40) and behavioral manifestations of anxiety at the interview (means = 1.13 vs. 0.40) were exhibited by the GAD group than by the DD group (both p's < .05). Conversely, higher symptoms of depressed mood (means = 3.40 vs. 2.03), psychomotor retardation (means = 1.53 vs. 1.03), and work impairment (means 3.20 vs. 2.20), as well as cognitions of helplessness (means = 2.33 vs. 1.57), hopelessness (means = 2.80 vs. 2.10), and worthlessness (means = 3.07 vs. 2.10), were exhibited by the DD group than by the GAD group (all p's $< .05$). Therefore, the depression symptoms were more discriminating than were the anxiety symptoms in the Albany sample.

Limitations. Apart from the limitations applying to any sample from a specialized referral base, including the Philadelphia CCT sample, one other potential shortcoming may apply to the Benshoof et al. (1990) findings. Nearly a third (27%) of their DD subjects (4 out of 15 cases) had secondary diagnoses of GAD. Moreover, because none of the DD subjects from the CCT sample had received a secondary diagnosis of GAD, or vice versa, the DD group from the Albany sample differed significantly from the DDs group in the CCT sample. Therefore, Benshoof et al. might have discriminated the groups more sharply with anxiety symptoms, had they not included DD subjects who also had GAD.

DISCUSSION

Despite the vast, accumulating literature dealing with anxiety and depression (see Chapter 1), the present chapter is the first published study to compare the specific presenting signs and symptoms of patients with GAD and patients with DD. In a systematic search, no published studies were found that had specifically compared these presenting signs and symptoms. Nevertheless, two previously unpublished evaluations of symptom overlap among GAD and DD patients have been presented.

1. *The discrimination of GAD and DD.* Contrary to any view that the anxiety and depression disorders are interchangeable, the findings of the CCT sample found that GAD and DD could be discriminated by both anxiety and depression, as well as by symptoms. Nevertheless, the results of the CCT sample and the Albany CSAD sample were not wholly consistent. Therefore, the present findings at most partially support the discrimination between these DSM-III or DSM-III-R disorders. In the following paragraphs, we now highlight several issues for future attention.

2. *Methodological issues.* Greater rigor is needed in future studies in selecting diagnostic and assessment procedures (see Chapter 10, this volume). First, studies are needed comparing GAD and DD patients diagnosed with psychometrically sound structured interviews; examples of such interviews are the ADIS-R and the SCID.

Second, such studies should use symptom measures that do not overlap in item content (Riskind et al., 1987). For example, the Hamilton Rating

Scale for Depression, as originally scored, contains numerous anxiety items; likewise, the Hamilton Anxiety Rating Scale contains several depression items. Of course, the crossover (and impurity) of item content accounts for a part of the correlation often found between measures of anxiety and depression (Riskind et al., 1987; Dobson, 1985; Gotlib, 1984; Tellegen, 1985). Nevertheless, the revised scoring system developed by Riskind et al. (1987) has reduced some of the overlap, so that the revised scores discriminate better between pure cases of GAD and DD than do the original Hamilton scales (e.g., for the revised scores, means for depression = 11.23 vs. 6.65, $p < .0001$; and for the original scores, means = 14.06 vs. 11.38, $p < .06$).

Assessment procedures could refine the indices used to measure symptoms. For example, Roth et al. (1972) reported that although episodic anxiety was associated with depression, persistent anxiety characterized anxiety disorders. Likewise, episodic depression appeared in anxiety disorders, whereas persistent depression characterized depression disorders. Therefore, refined indices might sharpen discrimination of GAD and DD.

Likewise, available data from the Hamilton scales fail to permit fine-grained analysis of the more discrete symptoms (e.g., muscle aches), because the Hamilton scales typically group such symptoms into larger units. Of course, symptom data obtained from existing data sets (but not yet coded for fine-grained analysis) could be recoded to analyze symptoms at the discrete level. Consequently, GAD and DD might be better discriminated by fine-grained analysis.

3. *Diagnostic issues: Heterogeneity of GAD and DD populations and comorbidity.* Are the presumed differences between the anxiety and depression disorders obtained over potential variations and subtypes of each category? This issue is relevant, because both GAD (Hoehn-Saric & McLeod, 1985) and DD (Akiskal, 1983) are heterogeneous disorders. For instance, Hoehn-Saric and McLeod (1985) have discriminated between one subtype of GAD patients who show muscle tension and autonomic arousal (e.g., elevation of heart rate, skin conductance) after the onset of stress, and another subtype of GAD patients who show only muscle tension. In all likelihood, the GAD patients without autonomic symptoms would be harder to distinguish from DD patients than the GAD patients with autonomic symptoms.

DD is divided into relevant subtypes based on onset patterns. In fact, Klein et al. (1988) found that early-onset (before age 25) DD was associated with more comorbid anxiety disorders than was late-onset (25 or after) DD. The findings of Klein et al. could imply that cases of GADs are harder to distinguish from early-onset cases of DD than from late-onset ones.

Therefore, we predict the highest overlap between cases of GAD and early-onset DD.

These differences in anxiety between early- and late-onset DD could also imply other differences in the nature of the disorders. One interpretation, for instance, is that *early*-onset DD produces greater impairment of social skills and coping skills (including cognitive ones) for managing the environment and anxiety; consequently, patients with early-onset DD may have higher anxiety because they have higher anxiety-related cognitions and less highly developed coping skills than do patients with late-onset DD. Future studies can examine (a) whether a practicing clinician can discriminate equivalently between GAD and early- and late-onset DD, and (b) early- and late-onset DD differ in their coping skills and cognitions.

Of course, as disorders, GAD and DD can occur concomitantly with each other as well as with other anxiety and depression disorders. When GADs and DDs are "impure" or mixed, they are likely to overlap more, and thus to be harder to discriminate. Nevertheless, our findings within the CCT sample suggest that discriminations achieved with pure groups can generalize to mixed groups, as long as they do not show overlap in GAD or DD.

Regarding comorbidity, the present findings provide some support that symptoms of dual or mixed anxiety–depression disorders are both more numerous and more severe than the symptoms of either of the pure disorders alone (e.g., Clark & Watson, 1990). Nevertheless, the CCT findings indicate that there is more than a single variant of mixed anxiety–depression. Indeed, the mixed GAD group exhibited higher anxiety symptoms, and higher depression on the revised Hamilton Rating Scale for Depression. They also had higher symptoms, for early-morning wakening and for weight loss, and higher anxiety-related cognitions on the Cognitions Checklist, than the mixed DD group. Consequently, mixed GAD was not interchangeable with mixed DD.

The co-occurrence rates, or comorbidity, of GAD and DD are also relevant evidence of the boundary between the disorders (see Chapter 6, this volume). Nevertheless, most current data are from cross-sectional studies. Thus, longitudinal studies are needed to explore the rates at which GAD shifts into DD, and vice versa, over time.

4. *Affective and cognitive variables that distinguish GAD from DD.* Affective and cognitive variables may help discriminate GAD and DD. Of course, such variables are likely to reflect overlap. Indeed, the factor of negative affect (comprised of feelings such as anger, fear, and sadness) appears to be common to both anxiety and depression. Nevertheless, the construct of low positive affect (comprised of feelings such as low interest, excitement,

and enjoyment) is widely regarded as an independent factor of affect. Moreover, low positive affect seems unique to anhedonia and depression (Tellegen, 1985; Clark, Beck, & Stewart, in press; Watson & Kendall, 1989; Clark & Watson, 1990; see also Chapter 8). It would be worth knowing whether negative affect and positive affect discriminate GAD and DD, in much the same way they discriminate MD and social phobia. It would also be worth knowing whether a more fine-grained analysis of specific discrete emotions (e.g., fear, anger) discriminates GAD and DD.

Particular attention must be directed to *anxiety*-related cognitive variables (e.g., worry) that distinguish GAD from DD. To be sure, depressive cognitions (e.g., hopelessness) have been successful in discriminating adequately between GAD and MD (Beck et al., 1987; Clark, et al., in press; Riskind, Castellon, & Beck, 1989). Nevertheless, anxiety-related cognitions closely related to worry, which is perhaps the crucial cognitive component of GAD (see Chapter 2, this volume), have failed to discriminate sufficiently between GAD and MD (e.g., Butler & Mathews, 1983; Greenberg & Beck, 1989). Of course, direct measures of worry have found that it is higher in GAD than in several other disorders (see Chapter 2). Nonetheless, moderate worry was found in 72% of a large sample of patients with MD (Fawcett & Kravitz, 1983). Therefore, some cognitive phenomena that are supposedly unique to anxiety may occur nonspecifically in both depression and anxiety.

The present CCT findings echo these outcomes. As expected, hopelessness and depressive cognitions on the Hamilton Rating Scale for Depression distinguished the subjects with pure GAD from the subjects with DD. Nevertheless, the measures that assessed variables related to worry—anxious cognitions on the Cognitions Checklist, and apprehensive expectations ("fears" and "anxious mood") on the Hamilton Anxiety Rating Scale—did not sufficiently distinguish subjects with pure GAD from subjects with pure DD. Indeed, the two groups had similar scores. Therefore, further evaluation is needed of any cognitive content specific to GAD and anxiety.

Indeed, a finer-grained approach to anxiety-related cognitions could be fruitful. For example, individuals with GAD and DD may worry in discriminable ways: Those with GAD perhaps worry about outcomes that loom or draw closer and are in a process of "becoming", yet still can be escaped from or avoided, whereas those with DD or MD may worry (or ruminate) about outcomes that they consider a matter of "being" which they are now powerless to change or avoid (for related research on a "looming" model, see Riskind, 1990). Of course, worry is only one of the cognitive phenomena in anxiety. Another aspect that could potentially discriminate GAD and DD is vigilance and scanning (e.g., MacLeod,

Mathews, & Tata, 1986). To be sure, neither the DSM-III-R criteria nor current anxiety scales seem to assess vigilance and scanning with sufficient behavioral detail. Therefore, we have recently developed a self-report questionnaire that is specifically intended to assess the behavioral aspects of vigilance (Riskind, Kaye, Lucas, Smith, & Hytree, 1990).

5. *Biological variables.* Physiological and biological factors could also discriminate GAD and DD (see Chapter 3, this volume). For example, several electroencephalographic sleep studies found that patients with GAD exhibited longer latencies to fall asleep and fewer awakenings than did patients with MD (e.g., Papadimitriou, Kerkhofs, Kempenaers, & Mendlewicz, 1988). Nevertheless, no sleep studies have compared patients with GAD and DD.

6. *Developmental antecedents and family studies.* Developmental, familial, and hereditary antecedents could also discriminate GAD and DD. Indeed, past studies of concordance rates in anxious patients have indicated that "anxiety neurosis" is influenced by hereditary factors (Torgersen, 1985). Nonetheless, our review found no equivalent studies for GAD. In a similar way, the Newcastle group (Roth et al., 1972) found a higher prevalence of neurotic illness and personality disturbance in first-degree relatives of patients with anxiety neurosis. Again, we located no similar studies of patients with GAD or DD. Of course, future studies could also compare the childhood environments of patients with GAD and DD, as well as their past history of stress and psychiatric disorders (e.g., Weissman, Leckman, Merikangas, Gammon, & Prusoff, 1984). Previous studies have indicated that anxiety and depression are preceded by different types of stressful life events (e.g., Smith & Allred, 1989; Finlay-Jones & Brown, 1981). Nonetheless, no prior studies have compared GAD and DD in this regard.

7. *Long-term course of the disorders.* Disorders have a future course as well as a past history. Earlier studies found that patients with anxiety neurosis (many having panic disorder) had more frequent and severe symptoms at follow-up than did patients with depression, who had the better global adjustment (Schapira, Roth, Kerr, & Gurney, 1972). Nevertheless, no studies have compared patients with GAD and DD in this respect. It is also likely that mortality rates might discriminate the disorders. Indeed, one prospective study of general population samples and psychiatric patients found that patients with a depression disorder (usually MD) experienced elevated mortality risks; however, patients with generalized anxiety had no increased risk (Murphy, Monson, Olivier, Sobol, & Leighton, 1987). Therefore, it would be interesting to evaluate whether patients with GAD and DD can be discriminated by their mortality risks and long-term course.

8. *Treatment response*. Differences in treatment response may also discriminate these two groups of patients (see Chapter 9). Indeed, the Newcastle group found that patients with depression versus "neurotic anxiety" (including panic) had different responses to tricyclic medications and electroconvulsive therapy (Gurney, Roth, Garside, Frith, & Schapira, 1972). Of course, recent studies have found little evidence for differential responses by anxious and depressed patients to pharmacological treatment (Johnstone et al., 1980). Nevertheless, it is possible that studies of patients with GAD and DD would find differences.

CONCLUSIONS

Our review of the literature found an astonishing hole in the published studies on anxiety and depression, none having previously evaluated GAD and DD patients for their overlap in symptoms. Nevertheless, this chapter has presented some evidence that there are individuals showing the classic signs of chronic anxiety, but not substantial depression. Likewise, there are individuals showing the classic signs of chronic depression, but not anxiety. Therefore, despite an overlap in symptoms, GAD and DD do not seem to be interchangeable disorders. Of course, our findings do not negate the possibility that GAD and DD are simply different points on a single continuum of affective disorder. Moreover, the groups seem to be better discriminated by depression than by anxiety, and the findings must all be replicated.

Of course, the symptoms of the patients with GAD and DD seem to parallel the widely proposed differences in the functions of anxiety and depression. Indeed, the patients with GAD seem to show many signs consistent with a chronic mobilization to prepare for threats (including higher autonomic arousal, cardiovascular symptoms, vigilance, and motor tension than patients with DD show). But the patients with DD, in contrast, seem to show many signs consistent with positive disengagement and conservation of energy (including higher hopelessness and depressed mood than patients with GAD, as well as suicidality and work difficulties). Nonetheless, the broader functions of anxiety and depression, and the adequacy of the DSM-IV categories, clearly need more probing attention.

REFERENCES

Akiskal, H. S. (1983). Dysthymic disorder: Psychopathology of proposed chronic depressive subtypes. *American Journal of Psychiatry, 140*, 11–20.
Barlow, D. H., Blanchard, E. B., Vermilyea, J. A., Vermilyea, B. B., & Di Nardo,

P. A. (1986). Generalized anxiety and generalized anxiety disorder: Description and reconceptualization. *American Journal of Psychiatry, 143,* 40–44.

Barlow, D. H., Di Nardo, P. A., Vermilyea, B. B., Vermilyea, J. A., & Blanchard, E. B. (1986). Co-morbidity and depression among the anxiety disorders: Issues in diagnosis and classification. *Journal of Nervous and Mental Disease, 174,* 63–72.

Beck, A. T., Brown, G., Steer, R. A., Eidelson, J. I., & Riskind, J. H. (1987). Differentiating anxiety and depression: A test of the content-specificity hypothesis. *Journal of Abnormal Psychology, 96,* 179–183.

Beck, A. T., Epstein, N., Brown, G., & Steer, R. A. (1988). An inventory for measuring clinical anxiety: Psychometric properties. *Journal of Consulting and Clinical Psychology, 56,* 893–897.

Beck, A. T., Kovacs, M., & Weissman, A. (1979). Assessment of suicidal intention: The Scale for Suicide Ideation. *Journal of Consulting and Clinical Psychology, 47,* 343–352.

Beck, A. T., Ward, C. H., Mendelson, M., Mock, J., Erbaugh, J. (1961). An inventory for measuring depression. *Archives of General Psychiatry, 4,* 561–571.

Beck, A. T., Weissman, A., Lester, D., & Trexler, L. (1974). The measurement of pessimism: The Hopelessness Scale. *Journal of Consulting and Clinical Psychology, 42,* 861–865.

Benshoof, B. B., Moras, K., Di Nardo, P. A., & Barlow, D. H. (1990). *A comparison of symptomatology in anxiety and depressive disorders.* Unpublished manuscript, Center for Stress and Anxiety Disorders, University of Albany, State University of New York.

Breier, A., Charney, D. S., & Heninger, G. R. (1985). The diagnostic validity of anxiety disorders and their relationship to depressive illness. *American Journal of Psychiatry, 142,* 787–797.

Butler, G., & Mathews, A. (1983). Cognitive processes in anxiety. *Advances in Behaviour Research and Therapy, 5,* 51–62.

Clancy, J., Noyes, R., Hoenk, P. R., & Slymen, D. J. (1979). Secondary depression in anxiety neurosis. *Journal of Nervous and Mental Disease, 166,* 846–850.

Clark, D. A., Beck, A. T., & Stewart, B. (in press). Cognitive specificity and positive–negative affectivity: Complementary or contradictory views on anxiety and depression? *Journal of Abnormal Psychology.*

Clark, L. A., & Watson, D. (1989). *Psychometric issues relevant to a potential DSM-IV category of mixed anxiety–depression.* Unpublished manuscript, DSM-IV Subgroup on Generalized Anxiety Disorder and Mixed Anxiety–Depression.

Dealy, R. S., Ishiiki, D. M., Avery, D. H., Wilson, L. G., & Dunner, D. L. (1981). Secondary depression in anxiety disorders. *Comprehensive Psychiatry, 22,* 612–617.

Di Nardo, P. A., & Barlow, D. H. (1988). *Anxiety Disorders Interview Schedule—Revised.* Albany: Center for Stress and Anxiety Disorders, University at Albany, State University of New York.

Di Nardo, P. A., & Barlow, D. H. (1990). Syndrome and symptom comorbidity in the anxiety disorders. In J. D. Maser & C. R. Cloninger (Eds.), *Comorbidity of anxiety and mood disorders.* Washington, DC: American Psychiatric Press.

Dobson, K. S. (1985). The relationship between depression and anxiety. *Clinical Psychology Review, 3,* 307–324.

Endicott, J., & Spitzer, R. L. (1978). A diagnostic interview: The Schedule for Affective Disorders and Schizophrenia. *Archives of General Psychiatry, 35,* 837–844.

Fawcett, J., & Kravitz, H. M. (1983). Anxiety syndromes and their relationship to depressive illness. *Journal of Clinical Psychiatry, 44,* 8–11.

Finlay-Jones, R., & Brown, G. W. (1981). Types of stressful events and the onset of anxiety and depressive disorders. *Psychological Medicine, 11,* 881–889.

Garvey, M., Cook, B., & Noyes, R., Jr. (1989). Comparison of major depressive patients with a predominantly sad versus anxious mood. *Journal of Affective Disorders, 17,* 183–187.

Gotlib, I. H. (1984). Depression and general psychopathology in university students. *Journal of Abnormal Psychology, 90,* 521–530.

Greenberg, M. S., & Beck, A. T. (1989. Depression versus anxiety: A test of the content-specificity hypothesis. *Journal of Abnormal Psychology, 98,* 9–13.

Gurney, C., Roth, M., Garside, R. F., Kerr, T. A., & Schapira, K. (1972). Studies in the classification of affective disorders: The relationship between anxiety states and depressive illness—II. *British Journal of Psychiatry, 121,* 162–166.

Hamilton, M. (1959). The assessment of anxiety states by rating. *British Journal of Medical Psychology, 32,* 50–55.

Hamilton, M. (1960). A rating scale for depression. *Journal of Neurology, Neurosurgery and Psychiatry, 23,* 56–61.

Hoehn-Saric, R., & McLeod, D. R. (1985). Generalized anxiety disorder. *Psychiatry Clinics of North America, 8,* 73–87.

Johnstone, E. C., Cunningham, O., Frith, C. D., McPherson, C. D., Reilly, G., & Gold, A. (1980). Neurotic illness and its response to anxiolytic and antidepressant medication. *Psychological Medicine, 10,* 321–329.

Klein, D. N., Taylor, E. B., Dickstein, S., & Harding, K. (1988). The early–late onset distinction in DSM-III-R dysthymia. *Journal of Affective Disorders, 14,* 25–33.

MacLeod, C., Mathews, A., & Tata, P. (1986). Attentional bias in emotional disorders. *Journal of Abnormal Psychology, 95,* 15–20.

Murphy, J. M., Monson, R. R., Olivier, D. C., Sobol, A. M., & Leighton, A. H. (1987). Affective disorders and mortality: A general population study. *Archives of General Psychiatry, 44,* 473–480.

Papadimitriou, G. N., Kerkhofs, M., Kempenaers, C., & Mendlewicz, J. (1988). EEG sleep studies in patients with generalized anxiety disorder. *Psychiatry Research, 26,* 183–190.

Parker, G., Blignault, I., & Manicavasagar, V. (1988). Neurotic depression: Delineation of symptom profiles and their relation to outcome. *British Journal of Psychiatry, 152,* 15–23.

Patich, D., & Crawford, G. *A multiple choice version of the WAIS Vocabulary subtest.* Unpublished manuscript, Clarke Institute of Psychiatry, Toronto.

Rapee, R. (1990). *Generalized anxiety disorder: Boundary issues with somatoform and psychophysiological disorders*. Unpublished manuscript, DSM-IV Subgroup on Generalized Anxiety Disorder and Mixed Anxiety–Depression.

Riskind, J. H. (1990). *The attribution of looming and increasing psychological proximity to threat predicts anxiety but not depression: Short-term prospective study of the "harm-looming" model*. Unpublished manuscript, George Mason University.

Riskind, J. H., Beck, A. T., Brown, G., & Steer, R. A. (1987). Taking the measure of anxiety and depression: Validity of the reconstructed Hamilton scales. *Journal of Nervous and Mental Disease, 22,* 474–478.

Riskind, J. H., Castellon, C. S., & Beck, A. T. (1989). Spontaneous causal explanations in unipolar depression and generalized anxiety: Content analyses of dysfunctional-thought diaries. *Cognitive Therapy and Research, 13,* 97–108.

Riskind, J. H., Kaye, C. A., Lucas, J., Smith, M., & Hytree, S. (1990, November). *Psychometric properties of a vigilance scale*. Paper presented at the annual meeting of the Association for Advancement of Behavior Therapy, San Francisco.

Rosenbaum, M. (1980). A schedule for assessing self-control behaviors: Preliminary findings. *Behavior Therapy, 11,* 109–121.

Roth, M., Gurney, C., Garside, R. F., & Kerr, T. A. (1972). Studies in the classification of affective disorders: The relation between anxiety states and depressive illness. *British Journal of Psychiatry, 121,* 147–161.

Roth, M., Mountjoy, C. Q., & Caetano, D. (1982). Further investigations into the relationship between depressive disorders and anxiety state. *Pharmacopsychiatry, 15,* 135–141.

Sanderson, W. C., & Barlow, D. H. (1990). A description of patients diagnosed with DSM-III-Revised generalized anxiety disorder. *Journal of Nervous and Mental Disease, 178,* 588–591.

Schapira, K., Roth, M., Kerr, T. A., & Gurney, C. (1972). The prognosis of affective disorders: The differentiation of anxiety states and depressive illnesses. *British Journal of Psychiatry, 121,* 175–181.

Smith, T. W., & Allred, K. D. (1989). Major life events in anxiety and depression. In P. C. Kendall & D. Watson (Eds.), *Anxiety and depression: Distinctive and overlapping features*. San Diego: Academic Press.

Spitzer, R. L., & Williams, J. B. W. (1983). *Instruction manual for the Structured Clinical Interview for DSM-III (SCID)*. New York: Biometrics Research Department, New York State Psychiatric Institute.

Spitzer, R. L., & Williams, J. B. W. (1985). Proposed revisions in the DSM-III classification of anxiety disorders based on research and clinical experience. In A. H. Tuma & J. Maser (Eds.), *Anxiety and the anxiety disorders*. Hillsdale, NJ: Erlbaum.

Spitzer, R. L., Williams, J. B. W., & Gibbon, M. (1987). *Structured Clinical Interview for DSM-III-R (SCID)*. New York: Biometrics Research Department, New York State Psychiatric Institute.

Tellegen, A. (1985). Structures of mood and personality and their relevance to assessing anxiety, with an emphasis on self report. In A. H. Tuma & J. D. Maser (Eds.), *Anxiety and the anxiety disorders*. Hillsdale, NJ: Erlbaum.

Torgersen, S. (1985). Hereditary differentiation of anxiety and affective neuroses. *British Journal of Psychiatry, 140,* 530–534.

Watson, D. A., & Kendall, P. C. (1989). Understanding anxiety and depression: Their relation to negative and positive affective states. In P. C. Kendall & D. Watson (Eds.), *Anxiety and depression: Distinctive and overlapping features.* San Diego: Academic Press.

Weissman, A., & Beck, A. T. (1978). *Development and validation of the Dysfunctional Attitude Scale: A preliminary investigation.* Paper presented at the meeting of the American Educational Research Association, Toronto.

Weissman, M. M., Leaf, P. L., Bruce, M. L., & Florio, L. (1988). The epidemiology of dysthymia in five communities: Rates, risks, comorbidity, and treatment. *American Journal of Psychiatry, 145,* 815–819.

Weissman, M. W., Leckman, J. F., Merikangas, K. R., Gammon, G. D., & Prusoff, B. A. (1984). Depression and anxiety disorders in parents and children. *Archives of General Psychiatry, 41,* 845–852.

Winokur, G. (1988). Anxiety disorders: Relationships to other psychiatric illness. *Psychiatric Clinics of North America, 11,* 287–293.

9

Pharmacotherapy of Generalized Anxiety Disorder

EDWARD SCHWEIZER
KARL RICKELS
University of Pennsylvania School of Medicine/University Hospital

Modern drug therapy of generalized anxiety disorder (GAD) has a 30-year history, beginning with the introduction of the first benzodiazepine (Bz), chlordiazepoxide, in 1960. The Bzs have been, in some ways, the victims of the success they enjoyed during the first 15 years after their introduction into medicine. The safety, patient acceptance, and rapid efficacy of this class of drugs led to widespread use that was frequently uncritical and indiscriminate. Too often Bzs have been prescribed as if they were a psychiatric form of antibiotic, and anxiety a "sore throat" that could be treated without regard to careful diagnosis. For example, the majority of depressed patients evaluated in primary care practices are prescribed a Bz as their sole form of treatment (Keller et al., 1982). Similarly, approximately one-third of the institutionalized elderly are prescribed Bzs for symptomatic relief of a mixed array of symptoms, including anxiety, depression, and insomnia (*National Disease and Therapeutic Index*, 1986; Mellinger, Balter, & Uhlenhuth, 1984).

In a series of surveys in the late 1970s and early 1980s, Mellinger and Balter (Mellinger et al., 1984; Mellinger & Balter, 1981) documented just how widespread the use of Bzs had become. From 10% to 12% of adults surveyed had taken a Bz in the past year, and fully 1.6% had taken a Bz daily for at least the past year. Recognition of the large extent of tranquilizer use, coupled with a growing public (Gordon, 1979; U.S. Senate, 1979) and professional (Lader, 1978; Hasday & Karch, 1981)

172

recognition of the problem of physical dependence and withdrawal, led to a backlash against Bzs. The backlash has taken the form of greater controls on prescribing (e.g., the New York State "triplicate" law); reduced per capita use; and, in the United Kingdom, calls for abandoning the use of Bzs altogether (Tyrer, 1984). The pharmaceutical industry, ever sensitive to a changing market, has responded by developing non-Bz anxiolytics such as buspirone (Rickels et al., 1982) and the as-yet-unmarketed gepirone (Csanalosi, Schweizer, Case, & Rickels, 1987) and ipsapirone (Borison, Albrecht, & Diamond, 1990) to treat anxious patients suffering from GAD, and by promoting recognition of panic anxiety as a distinct illness requiring aggressive Bz therapy.

Against this background, we briefly review the following issues relevant to the drug therapy of GAD: (1) What drugs have demonstrated efficacy and safety in the acute treatment of GAD? (2) When is acute drug therapy indicated, and which drug should be chosen? (3) When is maintenance drug therapy indicated, and how effective is it? and (4) What risks are associated with long-term drug therapy?

ACUTE DRUG THERAPY OF GAD

Two classes of compounds have demonstrated efficacy in the treatment of GAD (anxiety disorder without panic): the Bzs and the azapirones, to which may tentatively be added the tricyclic antidepressants.

Benzodiazepines

The most evidence for efficacy exists for the Bzs. Innumerable double-blind, controlled studies, conducted both before and after the publication of the *Diagnostic and Statistical Manual of Mental Disorders*, third edition (DSM-III), have confirmed the efficacy of the Bzs in the acute treatment of anxiety (Greenblatt, Shader, & Abernethy, 1983a, 1983b; Rickels & Schweizer, 1987; Rickels, 1978). About 70% of adequately treated patients respond significantly to Bz therapy, but only about 40% achieve remission of symptoms, while 30% are still at least mildly anxious (Rickels, 1978). In those patients who respond, treatment response is rapid (Downing & Rickels, 1985). Somatic and psychic symptoms of anxiety respond equally well. Yet we know little about how sustained the response to acute treatment is, what an adequate duration of acute (or, for that matter, chronic) treatment is, and whether or not one Bz offers advantages over any other. Many patients unimproved with Bz therapy may have never received an adequate daily dose, often because of lack of tolerance to the sedative and psychomotor-impairing side effects of Bzs. Others may have been misdiagnosed.

Many years ago, Rickels (1978) observed that early reports of sedation with diazepam were a significant predictor of anxiolytic response, probably serving as an indicator of appropriate minimum dose prescribed. Clear relationships have never been observed between improvement and either Bz plasma levels or prescribed daily dose, because most treatment-resistant patients are the ones who have been prescribed higher daily dosages; the majority of patients respond to daily dosages of 15–25 mg of diazepam or its equivalent levels (Rickels, Case, Downing, Dixon, & Fridman, 1984). Also, to our knowledge, there has never been a published study that characterizes or provides data on how to manage treatment-resistant GAD patients.

Since clinical response to Bz therapy is very rapid, with much of the improvement occurring in the first week (Downing & Rickels, 1985), a lack of response after 2–3 weeks of appropriately dosed Bz therapy suggests the need for a diagnostic reassessment. GAD is a common comorbid diagnosis with panic disorder, major depression, social phobia, and Axis II personality disorders (Noyes, Clancy, Hoenk, & Slymen, 1980; Barlow, Di Nardo, Vermilyea, Vermilyea, & Blanchard, 1986; Clancy, Noyes, Hoenk, & Slymen, 1978; Tyrer, Casey, & Gall, 1983; Koenigsberg, Kaplan, Gilmore, & Cooper, 1985; Weiss, Davis, Hedlund, & Cho, 1983; see also Chapter 6, this volume). Lack of adequate therapeutic response is commonly due to neglect of such co-occurring diagnoses.

Frequently, residual symptoms continue to be present, even in GAD patients who are responders to direct therapy. Again, there is little published research that directly addresses the issue, but it is our impression that chronic GAD often is associated with a high degree of concomitant Axis I psychopathology (particularly dysthymia or mild depressions), as well as Axis II psychopathology.

Yet about 50% of chronically anxious GAD patients in two studies, treated for 4–6 weeks with the Bzs, maintained their improvement for at least 2 weeks. In one study patients were followed up for only 2 weeks (Rickels, Fox, Greenblatt, Sandler, & Schless, 1988); in the other study patients were followed for 12 weeks while on placebo (Rickels, Case, Downing, & Winokur, 1983). One year later, however, of those patients who remained improved for 12 weeks, a significant number (63%) had again become anxious (Rickels, Case, Downing, & Fridman, 1986). These data thus support the notion that many GAD patients are chronically anxious, but the data also dispel the notion that all such patients are in need of continuous drug therapy. In fact, the majority of such patients may well benefit more from intermittent than from continuous drug therapy.

Treatment of this type of chronic GAD often meets with less satisfactory results, and frequently leads to chronic use of medication. Clearly, for a substantial number of GAD patients 6 weeks' worth of therapy is insufficient, but for whom it is insufficient we are unable to predict.

To date, there is no evidence that one Bz offers any therapeutic advantage over any other. All Bzs appear to achieve their clinical effect through agonist activity at the Bz–gamma-aminobutyric acid (GABA) receptor. This has been confirmed by studies in which the drug effect has been blocked by pretreatment with the selective Bz antagonist flumazenil (Brogden & Goa, 1988). Though there is no known therapeutic advantage for individual Bzs, there are pharmacokinetic differences in absorption, distribution, and receptor affinity, which might yield clinical differences in certain patients. Indeed, anecdotally we have observed patients to improve on one Bz when they have failed to respond to a comparable dose of another Bz.

We have reviewed the adverse effects of acute Bz therapy elsewhere (Rickels, Schweizer, & Lucki, 1987). Three often overlooked adverse effects deserve mention. First, subtle anterograde amnesia is occasionally observed, especially when high-potency Bzs are used (e.g., triazolam, alprazolam, or lorazepam). Second, there is an occasional paradoxical disinhibition of hostile and irritable behaviors; again, this is seen primarily with high-potency Bzs. (In the majority of anxious patients, Bzs reduce hostility.) Third, there is a detrimental effect of Bzs on delayed memory or memory consolidation; this has even been seen with an acute Bz dose in drug-naive patients (Lucki, Rickels, Giesecke, & Geller, 1987), as well as with chronic Bz users (Lucki, Rickels, & Geller, 1986).

In general, tolerance develops within a few weeks to most of the sedating and psychomotor-impairing side effects of Bzs, but very little to the anxiolytic effects (Lucki et al., 1986). The reduction in side effect severity with continued use is more pronounced for the Bzs than for the tricyclic antidepressants. Of interest is also the observation by Downing and Rickels (1981) that excessive coffee consumption decreases sedative complaints.

Azapirones

The azapirones are the second class of drugs that have demonstrated efficacy in the treatment of GAD. Buspirone is the only azapirone to date that has been marketed, though gepirone, ipsapirone, and other related compounds are presently under study. The azapirones do not act at the Bz–GABA receptor complex, nor do they appear to have much activity at sites other than serotonin (5-HT) receptor sites (Eison & Temple, 1986). As a result, the azapirones do not generally cause sedation, do not interact with alcohol or other sedatives, and do not appear to engender physical dependence or withdrawal with long-term use. This favorable clinical profile makes them an appealing treatment alternative to the Bzs.

Current speculation suggests that the azapirones achieve their clinical effect through a partial agonist activity at the 5-HT_1A receptor (Riblet, Taylor, Eison, & Stanton, 1982). Azapirones have activity at both the presynaptic and postsynaptic 5-HT_1A receptors, with the net effect that they appear to reduce 5-HT tone where a hyperserotonergic state exists, and to increase 5-HT tone where a hyposerotonergic state exists (Eison & Temple, 1986). This reciprocal ability to regulate serotonergic function is hypothesized to underlie the observed anxiolytic and possible antidepressant effects of these compounds.

Many studies have documented the anxiolytic effect of buspirone for patients suffering from GAD (Rickels et al., 1982; Cohn, Bowden, Fisher, & Rodos, 1986; Sussman, 1987). Preliminary research suggests similar efficacy for gepirone (Csanalosi et al., 1987) and ipsapirone (Borison et al., 1990). The existing research suggests that the azapirones generally take about 2–3 weeks before a clinical response is observed, so that p.r.n. (as-needed) use is not effective. The compounds have short elimination half-lives (less than 4 hours), so t.i.d. (thrice-daily) dosing is the common practice. Buspirone patients with prior Bz therapy were observed to respond less favorably to treatment than patients without such prior therapy (Schweizer, Rickels, & Lucki, 1986).

Several 5-HT_2 and 5-HT_3 antagonists are also being studied in GAD patients. Whether or not these compounds will exert anxiolytic activity in humans has not yet been determined, and placebo-controlled studies have not yet been reported upon.

Tricyclic Antidepressants

The final class of compounds that have demonstrated preliminary efficacy in the treatment of GAD are the tricyclic antidepressants. We are unaware of any published studies reporting the use of newer antidepressants, such as bupropion or fluoxetine, in the treatment of GAD.

The evidence for efficacy of antidepressants in GAD depends on a handful of studies, several conducted on patients with DSM-II diagnoses or a diagnosis of mixed anxiety–depression (Rickels et al., 1973; Rickels, Hesbacher, & Downing, 1970; Liebowitz et al., 1988). There is preliminary evidence, though, that tricyclic antidepressants may have efficacy in treating patients with more carefully screened GAD (Kahn et al., 1986; Rickels, Downing, & Schweizer, 1987).

INDICATIONS FOR DRUG THERAPY

When is drug therapy indicated? When is the agent of first choice a Bz versus an azapirone versus a tricyclic antidepressant? And what are predictors of good treatment response? These are only some of the questions to which clinicians seek answers.

At what point does GAD warrant formal treatment? The answer is both obvious and trivial: when the symptoms are sufficiently persistent and distressing that they interfere with normal functioning. By the DSM-III-R definition of GAD, with its combined symptom and duration criteria, *all cases of GAD probably deserve treatment*, either pharmacological or non-pharmacological. Yet population surveys suggest that only about 25% of persons with presumptive GAD are ever treated (Uhlenhuth, Balter, Mellinger, Cisin, & Clinthorne, 1983), and the vast majority of those who do get treatment never see a mental health specialist (Regier, Goldberg, & Taube, 1978).

When should drug therapy be recommended, and when should psychotherapy be? To our knowledge, there are no good, controlled studies that have compared drug therapy to psychotherapy for the treatment of GAD. As a result, the decision to treat with drugs is often based on the expertise of the physician being consulted, the preference of the patient, and the financial and time constraints that both are operating under. In regard to these constraints, there is every reason to believe that use of Bzs is cheaper and less labor-intensive than psychotherapeutic treatment, though Catalan, Gath, Edmonds, and Ennis (1984) have reported reduction in anxious symptoms after a surprisingly modest supportive intervention by primary care physicians.

On balance, there is much more accumulated empirical evidence to support the effectiveness of drugs than of various psychotherapies for the treatment of GAD. The Bzs are particularly effective for patients in need of short-term (1–2 weeks) or p.r.n. medication for anxiety. In contrast, buspirone appears to be most helpful to patients in need of chronic anxiolytic therapy.

There is evidence that prior use of Bzs effectively reduces the anxiolytic response to azapirones, perhaps as a result of lower patient satisfaction (Schweizer et al., 1986). Prominent insomnia, adrenergic symptoms, or a history of panic attacks also may reduce the likelihood of achieving a good therapeutic response to azapirones (Schweizer & Rickels, 1988; Sheehan, Raj, Sheehan, & Soto, 1990). Buspirone appears to increase firing in the locus ceruleus (Eison & Temple, 1986; Riblet et al., 1982) and so may even worsen adrenergic symptoms, which presumably contribute to its lack of sedation. Conversely, concomitant depressive symptoms argue against use of Bzs, though there is evidence that alprazolam may have antidepressant properties in its own right (Rickels, Chung, et al., 1987). Instead, one might wish to treat anxious patients who have significant concomitant levels of depression with an azapirone (i.e., buspirone) or with a tricyclic antidepressant.

MAINTENANCE DRUG THERAPY

As we have discussed elsewhere (Rickels & Schweizer, 1990), GAD is a frequently chronic condition associated with significant comorbidity, disability, and subjective distress. Within this clinical context, maintenance medication therapy becomes an option. Little research, though, has been conducted to assess the efficacy of such chronic anxiolytic drug therapy.

The few studies that have assessed relapse rates after acute treatment suggest that more such studies are badly needed. Rickels, Case, and Diamond (1980) conducted a 1-year follow-up study of anxious patients given a DSM-II diagnosis of anxiety neurosis, who were treated for 4 weeks with Bzs. They observed a relapse rate of 81% at follow-up. A longer duration of illness prior to entering treatment was found to be the best predictor of early relapse. In another study, Rickels, Case, Downing, and Fridman (1986) treated 138 GAD patients with diazepam for at least 6 weeks. A relapse rate of 63% was found at re-examination 1 year later. Approximately 50% of the patients, however, were symptom-free for at least 3 months after diazepam treatment of 6 weeks' duration was discontinued (Rickels et al., 1983). Similar improvement rates were maintained for at least 2 weeks in two other acute studies of 4 weeks' duration with chronic GAD patients (Rickels, Fox et al., 1988). Yet rebound anxiety after acute treatment with Bzs (particularly high-potency ones) is definitely a possibility and occurs in about 20% of patients (Rickels, Fox, et al., 1988). These follow-up results indicate that for many chronically anxious GAD patients, a more prolonged treatment period may be indicated. Yet empirical confirmation of the benefit of maintenance drug therapy for chronic GAD is almost nonexistent.

Few long-term studies have been conducted with anxiolytics in GAD patients, and most of these were designed primarily to establish the safety of a specific drug for regulatory purposes, rather than to explore long-term clinical benefits. To our knowledge, only two double-blind, well-controlled studies exist in the literature—one with diazepam (Rickels et al., 1983), and one with clorazapate and buspirone (Rickels, Schweizer,

Csanalosi, Case, & Chung, 1988). These studies were designed to assess the anxiolytic efficacy of the two Bzs and buspirone over a 6-month treatment period in GAD patients. Both studies also included in their design a double-blind substitution of placebo for the anxiolytic medication at the end of the chronic treatment period. The most important clinical finding of these two studies, confirmed by a similar prospective 8-month treatment study of panic disorder (Schweizer, Rickels, Weiss, & Zavodnick, 1991), was that tolerance did not appear to develop to the anxiolytic effect of the benzodiazepines. Patients reported continued effective anxiolysis without any tendency to escalate their daily dose of drug. Though drug therapy was found to be effective for 6–8 months, the above-mentioned studies were not designed to answer the question of how many patients would have been symptom-free had they stopped their medication earlier. One might estimate the percentage to be close to 50%, based on a study by Rickels et al. (1983), in which chronic GAD patients were treated for only 6 weeks with diazepam and then switched to placebo under double-blind conditions for 12 weeks. No prospective information based on well-designed clinical trials is available about maintenance use of Bzs or non-Bz anxiolytics in GAD patients for periods longer than 6 months.

A retrospective assessment of 119 Bz-dependent patients, who had been receiving a Bz for an average of 8 years, found no evidence of dose escalation (Rickels, Case, Schweizer, Swenson, & Fridman, 1986). Since many of these long-term Bz users reported rather high baseline levels of anxiety, despite current daily Bz use, some tolerance to the anxiolytic effect may have occurred after daily use of the drug for several years. These chronic users also had significantly more personality psychopathology and more depressive psychopathology than non-Bz-dependent anxious controls (Rickels, Schweizer, Case, & Greenblatt, 1990; Schweizer, Rickels, Case, & Greenblatt, 1990; Rickels, Schweizer, Case, & Garcia-Espana, 1988). Although it is only speculation, one may wonder whether in some patients Bz dependence may not be the consequence of inadequate therapy of GAD comorbidity, such as depression or panic, with a result that patients cling to a drug therapy that offers only partial control of their symptoms. We have reported recently (Rickels & Schweizer, 1990) on a pilot follow-up study of patients treated chronically with buspirone and clorazapate who were followed up at 40 months after discontinuing maintenance drug therapy. At the 40-month follow-up, there was significantly more anxiolytic use by patients treated for 6 months with clorazapate than by those treated for 6 months with the non-Bz anxiolytic buspirone. Sixty-five percent of clorazapate-treated patients continued on a Bz whereas none of the buspirone-treated patients did, $\chi^2 (2) = 10.1, p < .01$.

RISKS OF MAINTENANCE DRUG THERAPY

Benzodiazepines

The Bzs appear to be well suited in many ways for prolonged anxiolytic therapy. They are extremely effective and safe (Greenblatt et al., 1983a, 1983b; Woods, Katz, & Winger, 1987), and tolerance appears to develop rapidly (within weeks) to the sedative and psychomotor-impairing effects of the drugs. In addition, as mentioned above, little tolerance appears to develop to the anxiolytic effect. As a result, dose escalation of Bzs in therapeutically treated populations is an unusual event. Bzs also offer the advantage of an extremely large safety margin, and consequently a low potential for fatal overdose when taken alone. Finally, they appear to have a relatively low abuse potential (Woods et al., 1987).

However, these positive qualities have to be considered in light of the side effects of Bzs, such as their negative effects on memory and such acute, dose-related central nervous system (CNS) effects as drowsiness and lethargy. Potentiation of these effects by alcohol and other CNS depressants is another risk associated with Bz therapy. Considerable controversy surrounds the issue of chronic Bz therapy. The evidence is clear that Bzs do cause physical dependence after prolonged use in the vast majority of patients, and that such dependence is associated with withdrawal reactions (Rickels, Schweizer, et al., 1990; Schweizer et al., 1990; Woods et al., 1987; Busto et al., 1986). Thus for maintenance therapy, intermittent rather than continuous therapy is recommended.

The risk of adverse medical effects from chronic Bz use has not been systematically assessed. Despite the lack of published information on this topic, significant medical complications from chronic Bz use seem unlikely at this point, given the large number of patients over the last 30 years who have received them. Whether chronic use may cause detrimental cognitive or psychomotor effects that persist after discontinuation of the drug is still unresolved. Petursson, Gudjonsson, and Lader (1983), for example, reported persistent psychomotor deficits caused by chronic Bz use, but Lucki et al. (1986) were unable to confirm these findings.

A question has been raised concerning whether chronic Bz use might be associated with greater ventricular—brain ratios on computed tomography scans. Pilot studies have both supported (Lader, Ron, & Petursson, 1984; Perera, Powell, & Jenner, 1987) and contradicted (Rickels, 1985; Poser, Poser, Roscher, & Argyrakis, 1983) this tentative finding, which may well be due to factors other than Bz treatment, such as concurrent alcohol use. Finally, whether long-term use of Bzs, in some unsuspected way, impairs a patient's general ability to cope with new situations or stresses is a topic of great clinical importance. One recently published pilot study in human volunteers suggest that such impairment may occur (Jensen, Hutchings, & Poulsen, 1989). However, similar findings have not yet been reported for patients receiving Bzs for long periods.

Nevertheless, one may speculate that the constant use of Bz tranquilizers may keep patients from sharpening their coping skills; they may come to rely instead on medication for anxiety relief. It is for this reason that good clinicians encourage patients to improve their coping skills while Bzs keep their anxiety at a manageable level, in the hope that the patients will eventually be able to cope with life stresses without using medication (see Chapter 10, this volume).

Azapirones

In the aggregate, patients report slightly less satisfaction from acute therapy with buspirone than from therapy with Bzs. The higher attrition rate may be due to the history of prior Bz use (Schweizer et al., 1986) or to a lack of subtle euphoriant effects. It also may be due to a somewhat lower efficacy in GAD patients; this lower efficacy may result from the lack of response of patients suffering from GAD who also have intermittent panic attacks. Despite somewhat lower patient satisfaction with acute treatment, there is much to recommend the use of buspirone for chronic anxiolytic therapy. The 6-month prospective study that has been reported above found that no tolerance developed to the anxiolytic effect of buspirone. In addition, buspirone appears to be extremely safe, with no prominent impairment of psychomotor functions (Lader, 1982; Moskowitz & Smiley, 1982) and an apparent lack of physical dependence and abuse liability (Rickels, Schweizer, Csanalosi, et al., 1988; Cole, Orzack, Beake, Bird, & Bar-Tal, 1982) with chronic use. Moreover, there is preliminary evidence that buspirone may possess antidepressant properties, which would also recommend it for use in GAD (Schweizer, Amsterdam, Rickels, Kaplan, & Droba, 1986; Rickels, Amsterdam, et al., 1990; Robinson et al., 1990). This is especially important since many chronically anxious GAD patients also suffer from significant concomitant levels of depression, and many develop full-fledged major depressive episodes as one of the sequelae of their chronic illness (see Chapter 6, this volume). Further research, however, is necessary to fully establish buspirone's role in the long-term management of depression.

Imipramine

There are no available studies concerning the efficacy of maintenance tricyclic antidepressant therapy in the treatment of chronic GAD. Clearly, the tricyclic antidepressants are less safe and less well tolerated than either the Bzs or buspirone, and tend to produce notable anticholinergic side effects that many anxious patients are unwilling to endure. Yet the lack of dependence liability and the likelihood of prophylaxis of intercurrent depression recommend these agents as potential treatment options for the maintenance therapy of chronic GAD.

CONCLUSION

The research on the pharmacotherapy of GAD has been relatively neglected, compared to the effort devoted to pharmacotherapy of panic disorder or major depression. The effectiveness of Bzs and the azapirones for acute treatment is well documented, but clinicians wishing to make informed treatment decisions are confronted with gaps in empirical knowledge when it comes to choice of drug, optimal duration of acute therapy, rates of relapse after acute therapy, indications, benefits and duration of maintenance therapy, and so forth. It should be emphasized that this absence of well-designed, prospective research extends to the nondrug therapies for GAD, where there is even less information available (see Chapter 10 for a review).

GAD is, next to simple phobia, the most prevalent anxiety disorder. In the guise of "anxiety neurosis," it has been the paradigm of neuroses since Freud's time. It is perhaps ironic, then, that it has fallen into such disuse that psychiatrists appear to make the diagnosis only rarely. Little National Institute of Mental Health research is conducted on it, and the majority of GAD patients are treated by nonpsychiatric clinicians. This is a state of affairs that appears unlikely to change any time soon.

REFERENCES

Barlow, D. H., Di Nardo, P. A., Vermilyea, B. B., Vermilyea, J. A., & Blanchard, E. B. (1986). Co-morbidity and depression among the anxiety disorders: Issues in diagnosis and clarification. *Journal of Nervous and Mental Disease*, *174*, 63–72.

Borison, R. L., Albrecht, J. W., & Diamond, L. (1990). Efficacy and safety of a putative anxiolytic agent: Ipsapirone. *Psychopharmacology Bulletin*, *26*, 207–210.

Brogden, R. N., & Goa, K. L. (1988). Flumazenil: A preliminary review of its benzodiazepine antagonist properties, intrinsic activity and therapeutic use. *Drugs*, *35*, 449–467.

Busto, U., Seller, E. M., Naranjo, C. A., Cappell, H., Sanchez-Craig, M., & Sykora, K. (1986). Withdrawal reaction after long-term therapeutic use of benzodiazepines. *New England Journal of Medicine*, *315*, 854–859.

Catalan, J., Gath, D., Edmonds, G., & Ennis, J. (1984). The effects of nonprescribing of anxiolytics in general practice. *British Journal of Psychiatry, 144*, 593–610.

Clancy, J., Noyes, R., Hoenk, P. R., & Slymen, D. J. (1978). Secondary depression in anxiety neurosis. *Journal of Nervous and Mental Disease, 166*, 846–850.

Cohn, J. B., Bowden, C. L., Fisher, J. G., & Rodos, J. J. (1986). Double-blind comparison of buspirone and clorazepate in anxious outpatients. *American Journal of Medicine, 80* (suppl. 3b), 10–16.

Cole, J. O., Orzack, M. H., Beake, B., Bird, M., & Bar-Tal, Y. (1982). Assessment of the abuse liability of buspirone in recreational drug users. *Journal of Clinical Psychiatry, 43*(12 sec. 2), 69–74.

Csanalosi, I., Schweizer, E., Case, W. G., & Rickels, K. (1987). Gepirone in anxiety: A pilot study. *Journal of Clinical Psychopharmacology, 7*, 31–33.

Downing, R. W., & Rickels, K. (1981). Coffee consumption, cigarette smoking and the reporting of drowsiness in anxious patients treated with benzodiazepines or placebo. *Acta Psychiatrica Scandinavica, 64*, 398–408.

Downing, R. W., & Rickels, K. (1985). Early treatment response in anxious outpatients treated with diazepam. *Acta Psychiatrica Scandinavica, 72*, 522–528.

Eison, A. S., & Temple, D. L. (1986). Buspirone: Review of its pharmacology and current perspectives on its mechanism of action. *American Journal of Medicine, 80*(suppl. 3B), 1–9.

Gordon, B. (1979). *I'm dancing as fast as I can.* New York: Harper & Row.

Greenblatt, D. J., Shader, R. I., & Abernethy, D. R. (1983a). Current status of benzodiazepines: Part I. *New England Journal of Medicine, 309*, 354–398.

Greenblatt, D. J., Shader, R. I., & Abernethy, D. R. (1983b). Current status of benzodiazepines: Part II. *New England Journal of Medicine, 309*, 410–416.

Hasday, J. D., & Karch, F. E. (1981). Benzodiazepine prescribing in a family medicine center. *Journal of the American Medical Association, 246*, 1321–1325.

Jensen, H. H., Hutchings, B., & Poulson, J. C. (1989). Conditioned emotional responding under diazepam: A psychological study of state dependent learning. *Psychopharmacology, 98*, 392–397.

Kahn, R. J., McNair, D. M., Lipman, R. S., Covi, L., Rickels, K., Downing, R., Fisher, S., & Frankenthaler, L.M. (1986). Imipramine and chlordiazepoxide in depressive and anxiety disorders: II. Efficacy in anxious outpatients. *Archives of General Psychiatry, 43*, 79–85.

Keller, M. B., Klerman, G. L., Lavori, P. W., Fawcett, J. A., Coryell, W., & Endicott, J. (1982). Treatment received by depressed patients. *Journal of the American Medical Association, 248*, 1848–2855.

Koenigsberg, H. W., Kaplan, R. D., Gilmore, M. M., & Cooper, A. M. (1985). The relationship between syndrome and personality disorder in DSM-III: Experience with 2,462 patients. *American Journal of Psychiatry, 142*, 207–212.

Lader, M. H. (1978). Benzodiazepines—the opium of the masses? *Neuroscience, 3*, 159–165.

Lader, M. H. (1982). Psychological effects of buspirone. *Journal of Clinical Psychiatry, 43* (12, sec. 2), 62–67.

Lader, M. H., Ron, M., & Petursson, H. (1984). Computerized axial brain tomography in long-term benzodiazepine users. *Psychological Medicine*, *14*, 203–206.

Liebowitz, M. R., Fyer, A. J., Gorman, J. M., Campeas, R. B., Sandberg, D. P., Hollander, E., Pappa, L. A., & Klein, D. F. (1988). Tricyclic therapy of the DSM-III anxiety disorders: A review with implications for further research. *Journal of Psychiatric Research*, *22* (1, Suppl.), 7–31.

Lucki, I., Rickels, K., & Geller, A. M. (1986). Chronic use of benzodiazepines and psychomotor and cognitive test performance. *Psychopharmacology*, *88*, 426–433.

Lucki, I., Rickels, K., Giesecke, M. A., & Geller, A. (1987). Differential effects of the anxiolytic drugs, diazepam and buspirone, on memory function. *British Journal of Clinical Pharmacology*, *23*, 207–211.

Mellinger, G. D., & Balter, M. B. (1981). Prevalence and patterns of use of psychotherapeutic drugs: Results from a 1979 national survey of American adults. In G. Tognoni, C. Bellantuono, & M. H. Lader (Eds.), *Epidemiological impact of psychotropic drugs*. New York: Elsevier/North-Holland.

Mellinger, G. D., Blater, M. B., & Uhlenhuth, E. H. (1984). Prevalence and correlates of the long-term regular use of anxiolytics. *Journal of the American Medical Association*, *251*, 375–379.

Moskowitz, H., & Smiley, A. (1982). Effects of chronically administered buspirone and diazepam on driving-related skills performance. *Journal of Clinical Psychiatry*, *43* (12, Sec. 2), 45–55.

National disease and therapeutic index. (1986). Ambler, PA: IMS.

Noyes, R., Clancy, J., Hoenk, P. R., & Slymen, D. J. (1980). The prognosis of anxiety disorders. *Archives of General Psychiatry*, *37*, 173–178.

Perera, K. H. M., Powell, T., & Jenner, F. A. (1987). Computerized axial tomographic studies following long-term use of benzodiazepines. *Psychological Medicine*, *17*, 775–777.

Petursson, H., Gudjonsson, G. H., & Lader, M. H. (1983). Psychometric performance during withdrawal from long-term benzodiazepine treatment. *Psychopharmacology*, *81*, 345–349.

Poser, W., Poser, S., Roscher, D., & Argyrakis, A. (1983). Do benzodiazepines cause cerebral atrophy? [Letter]. *Lancet*, *i*, 715.

Regier, D. A., Goldberg, I. D., & Taube, C. A. (1978). The de facto U.S. mental health services system: A public health perspective. *Archives of General Psychiatry*, *35*, 685–693.

Riblet, L. A., Taylor, D. P., Eison, M. S., & Stanton, H. C. (1982). Pharmacology and neurochemistry of buspirone. *Journal of Clinical Psychiatry*, *43* (12, Sec. 2), 11–16.

Rickels, K. (1978). Use of antianxiety agents in anxious outpatients. *Psychopharmacology*, *58*, 1–17.

Rickels, K. (1985). Clinical management of benzodiazepine dependence [Letter]. *British Medical Journal*, *291*, 1649.

Rickels, K., Amsterdam, J., Clary, C., Hassman, J., London, J., Puzzuoli, G., & Schweizer, E. (1990). Buspirone in depressed outpatients: A controlled study.

Psychopharmacology Bulletin, 26, 163–167.

Rickels, K., Case, W. G., & Diamond, L. (1980). Relapse after short-term drug therapy in neurotic outpatients. *International Pharmacopsychiatry, 15,* 186–192.

Rickels, K., Case, W. G., Downing, R. W., Dixon, R., & Fridman, R. (1984). Diazepam and desmethyldiazepam plasma concentrations in chronic anxious outpatients. *Pharmacopsychiatry, 17,* 44–49.

Rickels, K., Case, W. G., Downing, R. W., & Fridman, R. (1986). One-year follow-up of anxious patients treated with diazepam. *Journal of Clinical Psychopharmacology, 6,* 32–36.

Rickels, K., Case, W. G., Downing, R. W., & Winokur, A. (1983). Long-term diazepam therapy and clinical outcome. *Journal of the American Medical Association, 250,* 767–771.

Rickels, K., Case, W. G., Schweizer, E. E., Swenson, C., & Fridman, R. (1986). Low-dose dependence in chronic benzodiazepine users: A preliminary report on 119 patients. *Psychopharmacology Bulletin, 22,* 407–415.

Rickels, K., Chung, H. R., Csanalosi, I., Horowitz, A. M., London, J., Wiseman, K., Kaplan, M., & Amsterdam, J. D. (1987). Alprazolam, diazepam, imipramine and placebo in outpatients with major depression. *Archives of General Psychiatry, 44,* 862–866.

Rickels, K., Csanalosi, I., Chung, H. R., Case, W. G., Pereira-Ogan, J. A., & Weise, C. C. (1973). Amitriptyline, diazepam, and phenobarbital sodium in depressed outpatients. *Journal of Nervous and Mental Disease, 157,* 442–451.

Rickels, K., Downing, R. W., & Schweizer, E. (1987, May). *Antidepressants in generalized anxiety disorder.* Paper presented at the annual meeting of the American Psychiatric Association, Chicago.

Rickels, K., Fox, I. L., Greenblatt, D. J., Sandler, K. R., & Schless, A. (1988). Clorazepate and lorazepam: Clinical improvement and rebound anxiety. *American Journal of Psychiatry, 145*(3), 312–317.

Rickels, K., Hesbacher, P., & Downing, R. W. (1970). Differential drug effects in neurotic depression. *Diseases of the Nervous System, 31,* 468–475.

Rickels, K., & Schweizer, E. (1987). Current pharmacotherapy of anxiety and panic. In H. Y. Meltzer (Ed.), *Psychopharmacology: The third generation of progress.* New York: Raven Press.

Rickels, K., & Schweizer, E. (1990). The clinical course and long-term management of generalized anxiety disorder. *Journal of Clinical Psychopharmacology, 10,* 101S–110S.

Rickels, K., Schweizer, E., Case, G. W., & Garcia-Espana, F. (1988). Benzodiazepine dependence, withdrawal severity, and clinical outcome: Effects of personality. *Psychopharmacology Bulletin, 24,* 415–420.

Rickels, K., Schweizer, E., Case, W. G., & Greenblatt, D. J. (1990). Long-term therapeutic use of benzodiazepines. *Archives of General Psychiatry, 47,* 899–907.

Rickels, K., Schweizer, E., Csanalosi, I., Case, W. G., & Chung, H. (1988). Long-term treatment of anxiety and risk of withdrawal: Prospective comparison of clorazepate and buspirone. *Archives of General Psychiatry, 45,* 444–450.

Rickels, K., Schweizer, E., & Lucki, I. (1987). Benzodiazepine side effects. In R. E. Hales & A. J. Frances (Eds.), *American Psychiatric Association annual review* (Vol. 6). Washington, DC: American Psychiatric Press.

Rickels, K., Wiseman, K., Norstad, N., Singer, M., Stoltz, D., Brown, A., & Danton, J. (1982). Buspirone and diazepam in anxiety: A controlled study. *Journal of Clinical Psychiatry, 43* (12, Sec. 2), 81–86.

Robinson, D. S., Rickels, K., Feighner, J., Fabre, L. F., Gammans, R. E., Shrotriya, R. C., Alms, D. R., Andary, J. J., & Messina, M. E. (1990). Clinical effects of the 5-HT1a partial agonists in depression: A composite analysis of buspirone in the treatment of depression. *Journal of Clinical Psychopharmacology, 10,* 67S–76S.

Schweizer, E., Amsterdam, J., Rickels, K., Kaplan, M., & Droba, M. (1986). Open trial of buspirone in the treatment of major depressive disorder. *Psychopharmacology Bulletin, 22,* 183–185.

Schweizer, E., & Rickels, K. (1988). Buspirone in the treatment of panic disorder: A controlled pilot comparison with clorazepate. *Journal of Clinical Psychopharmacology, 8,* 303.

Schweizer, E., Rickels, K., Case, W. G., & Greenblatt, D. J. (1990). Long-term therapeutic use of benzodiazepines. *Archives of General Psychiatry, 47,* 908–915.

Schweizer, E., Rickels, K., & Lucki, I. (1986). Resistance to the anti-anxiety effect of buspirone in patients with a history of benzodiazepine use. *New England Journal of Medicine, 314,* 719–720.

Schweizer, E., Rickels, K., Weiss, S., Zavodnick, S. (1991). Maintenance drug treatment for panic disorder I. Results of a prospective, placebo-controlled comparison of alprazolam and imipramine.

Sheehan, D., Raj, A. B., Sheehan, H., & Soto, S. (1990). Is buspirone effective for panic disorder? *Journal of Clinical Psychopharmacology, 10,* 3–11.

Sussman, N. (1987). Treatment of anxiety with buspirone. *Psychiatric Annals, 17,* 114–120.

Tyrer, P. J. (1984). Benzodiazepines on trial. *British Medical Journal, 288,* 1101–1102.

Tyrer, P. J., Casey, P., & Gall, J. (1983). Relationship between neurosis and personality disorder. *British Journal of Psychiatry, 142,* 404–408.

Uhlenhuth, E. H., Balter, M. B., Mellinger, G. D., Cisin, I. H., & Clinthorne, J. (1983). Symptom checklist syndromes in the general population: Correlations with psychotherapeutic drug use. *Archives of General Psychiatry, 40,* 1167–1173.

U.S. Senate, Subcommittee on Health and Scientific Research, Committee on Human Resources. (1979, September 10). *The use and abuse of Valium, Librium and other benzodiazepine tranquilizers.* Transcript of hearing.

Weiss, J. M. A., Davis, D., Hedlund, J. L., & Cho, D. W. (1983). The dysphoric psychopath: A comparison of 524 cases of antisocial personality disorder with matched controls. *Comprehensive Psychiatry, 24,* 355–369.

Woods, J. H., Katz, J., & Winger, G. (1987). Abuse liability of benzodiazepines. *Pharmacological Reviews, 39,* 251–419.

10

Developing Psychological Treatments for Generalized Anxiety Disorder

GILLIAN BUTLER
Warneford Hospital, Headington, Oxford

RICHARD G. BOOTH
University of British Columbia

Attempting to grapple with issues surrounding generalized anxiety disorder (GAD) can all too easily lead to some feelings associated with the condition itself. The inconsistent research findings, treatment obstacles, and diffuse nature of the disorder can bring on very similar feelings of being demoralized, confused, and overwhelmed. It is hardly coincidental that there has been less research on this than on any of the other anxiety disorders, and that a relatively large proportion of these patients have responded rather poorly to psychological treatment. The way forward that we adopt in this chapter is, on the one hand, to examine a specific set of research findings that will act as a guide, and, on the other, to use clinical impressions to speculate (at times with some liberty) on their conclusions. The aim is to discuss some of the important issues relating to treatment, rather than to provide a comprehensive review of outcome studies. Such an approach is appropriate, inasmuch as it reflects what seem to be two critical qualities for therapists dealing with this disorder: clarity and creativity. We argue that these characteristics may be critical to the success of any therapeutic approach to the treatment of GAD.

TWO TREATMENT OUTCOME STUDIES FOR GAD

We propose at the outset to review two studies carried out in Oxford that focused on the treatment of GAD. The rest of the chapter draws on their findings, links them to clinical impressions, and (in the "Discussion" section) combines these two sources of information in an attempt to identify possible sources of treatment effectiveness. These are then considered in the context of some of the other recent literature in the area.

The two studies to be reviewed were developed out of sustained attempts to try out principles and techniques of behavior therapy in more testing spheres than on the simple phobias for which they had proved so successful (Jannoun, Oppenheimer, & Gelder, 1982; Butler, Cullington, Munby, Amies, & Gelder, 1984). The particular interest was in whether such techniques as relaxation and exposure would be similarly effective for more generalized fears, such as social phobia and GAD. The techniques might be expected to have limitations with such fears. Though relaxation techniques have been widely used and seem to be beneficial in the short term, their lasting effects have not been so well supported. Of course, the techniques may not have been effectively taught, and patients appear to practice less as time goes on. More significantly however, relaxation clearly fails to deal directly with two vital components of anxiety disorders: cognitions and avoidance behavior. Exposure is certainly effective with regard to the latter, though even in that sphere it is not without its own important difficulties (see Butler, 1985). In social phobia, for instance, a range of subtle kinds of avoidance makes habituation to feared situations much less likely: Many patients report that they use a kind of "internal avoidance," which prevents full engagement in anxiety-provoking activities despite apparent exposure. Subtle kinds of avoidance also occur in GAD. For example, patients report avoiding doing anything that might exacerbate their symptoms, or anything that might make them worry, without being able to predict when this might be necessary or to describe exactly what their fear would lead them to avoid.

Such limitations led to the development of a more comprehensive package—a variety of techniques based on the idea, similar to that of Suinn and Richardson (1971) for "anxiety management training," that it is possible to teach generalizable skills for coping with anxiety states. The anxiety management (AM) package that was developed for social phobia included relaxation, distraction, and a simple but individualized cognitive component focusing on the identification of and response to each person's specific thoughts. The results were encouraging, with exposure and AM being more effective than a combination of exposure and a nonspecific associative therapy (Butler et al., 1984). It was uncertain whether AM was acting by encouraging exposure or through specific effects of its own, but such questions needed no longer to be kept to the area of social phobias. At this point it was decided to try out a similar package on patients with GAD.

The first of the Oxford GAD studies described here (Butler, Cullington, Hibbert, Klimes, & Gelder, 1987) was quite straightforward. Since it was felt that so little was known about GAD, a waiting-list control group was compared with a group receiving AM (a version of the package that had been used with social phobia, expanded so as to include exposure and procedures to build confidence). AM proved to have a substantial effect not only on measures of anxiety, but also on those of depression and of the frequency of panic attacks. These changes were replicated almost exactly when patients in the waiting-list group completed treatment. At the same time an opportunity was taken to make various observations about patients with GAD (Butler, Gelder, Hibbert, Cullington, & Klimes, 1987), three of which are mentioned here.

1. Consistent with other evidence (Beck, Laude, & Bohnert, 1974; Hibbert, 1984; Rapee, 1985), there was a pattern of cognitions that was peculiar to GAD, though it had some overlap with those of other anxiety disorders. In addition, compared (for example) to depressed patients, those with GAD found it easy to identify cognitions associated with anxiety. Their thoughts reflected perceived vulnerability, characterized by enhanced perception of threat (e.g., "Something will go wrong," "I might get ill") and perceived lack of resources for dealing with it (e.g., "I shan't be able to cope," "There's nothing I can do," "This is more than I can manage").

2. On the other hand, at variance with other reports in the literature was the finding that nonphobic, generally anxious patients clearly described both situational anxiety and avoidance. The feared situations were varied; this diffuse pattern contrasted with the more focused avoidance of a smaller number of situations by phobic patients. In addition, avoidance often took subtle forms. Examples included avoiding thinking about problems, feelings, or fears; avoiding taking on additional tasks; and avoiding doing anything that might provoke distressing affect in others, such as anger or irritation.

3. A third finding was that patients who were most demoralized responded least well, especially if their resources for coping were limited or underused (Butler & Anastasiades, 1988). Although we lacked comparative data concerning the relative levels of demoralization in patients with GAD and others, it was striking that demoralization was very common in this population of patients with severe and persistent GAD (see below).

A natural progression was to examine some of the questions that had been left unanswered in this first study by comparing two treatments. First, it was of interest to find out how a direct behavioral approach including exposure would fare without a cognitive element, as avoidance clearly played a greater part in the disorder than had originally been supposed. This behavioral treatment also included relaxation and procedures to build confidence. Second, it was decided to use the cognitive–behavioral model described by Beck (Beck, Rush, Shaw, & Emery, 1979; Beck, Emery, & Greenberg, 1985), to see whether this would produce results superior to the much less elaborate cognitive strategies used within the coping model that characterized AM. A comparison of behavior therapy (BT) with cognitive–behavior therapy (CBT) offered a whole set of intriguing possibilities; it permitted separate analysis of cognitive and behavioral approaches to the problem, both of which might have contributed to the original success of AM.

The central findings of the study (Butler, Fennell, Robson, & Gelder, 1991), and the ones with which the following discussion should be consistent, were as follows:

1. Those patients in the BT group who completed treatment improved significantly on all but one measure of anxiety and maintained this improvement for the following 6 months.

2. There was a consistent pattern of change supporting the superiority of CBT over BT. This was evident not only in change on anxiety measures, but also in the absence of attrition and in the greater amount of cognitive change, the differences on the latter tending to increase with time after treatment.

3. There was support for the predictions that CBT would reduce depression as well as anxiety in patients who had both types of symptoms, and that patients in the CBT group would be more resistant to early relapse.

We propose to offer some explanation for these results in the "Discussion" section. This explanation is based on two sources: observations concerning the nature of GAD, and a more detailed analysis of the content of the cognitive-behavioral therapy that was in this instance so successful. According to stringent criteria, CBT led to clinically significant change in 42% of patients 6 months after treatment had ended, compared with only 5% after BT.

QUESTIONS POSED BY THE NATURE OF GAD

Without question, discussion on GAD has been greatly facilitated by the new definition of the disorder in the *Diagnostic and Statistical Manual of Mental Disorders*, third edition, revised (DSM-III-R; American Psychiatric Association, 1987). Patients with GAD are no longer in the "ragbag" category, including all those people who may be difficult to place in the other anxiety disorders. The strengths of the new definition stem from its clear focus on the essential feature of "anxious expectation" or worry, and the insistence on a minimum duration of 6 months (see Chapter 5, this volume).

It is of great help for purposes of diagnosis and research to have concise criteria for being a long-standing worrier, but some aspects of GAD are overlooked in the new definition. First, although it makes for clarity to define GAD in terms of worry about "two or more" life circumstances, this fails to make clear just how rare it is to worry about only two things. About two-thirds of the people with GAD in our study of BT versus CBT (Butler et al., 1991) said that they "had always been worriers," and that their worries had ranged over a great variety of concerns. Second, worry is a useful concept (as Borkovec and his colleagues are well aware), but we are only beginning to understand exactly what worry is and what it does (see Borkovec, Shadick, & Hopkins, Chapter 2, this volume; Borkovec, 1985; York, Borkovec, Vasey, & Stern, 1987; Borkovec & Hu, 1990; Borkovec & Inz, 1990). The content of worry often changes; physiological symptoms vary; the distress that it causes fluctuates and appears to be unpredictable; and it is not associated with the consistent, situation-specific avoidance found in phobic anxiety. Third, it is important not to ignore the consequences of having such a problem for a long period of time. In GAD two common secondary problems, depression and social anxiety, are easily recognizable in terms of diagnostic categories; a third problem, that of demoralization, may be more common still. "Demoralization" has not yet been precisely defined, but the constellation of symptoms becomes easy to recognize when one is treating GAD. It may include fatigue and withdrawal from demanding or pleasurable activities, loss of confidence and of self-esteem, and an acceptance of the status quo that verges on a nondepressed kind of hopelessness about the possibility of change. When asked to rate on a scale of 0–8 how demoralized they felt, only three patients in the Butler et al. (1991) study (about 7%) gave a rating below the midpoint of the scale, and the mean score of the remaining 93% was 6.2; that is, they rated themselves as being *very* demoralized.

If a treatment could focus on worry, anxious cognitions, avoidance, physical tension, and the secondary symptoms of depression and withdrawal, *and* could also tackle this problem of demoralization, then it should certainly be expected to do well. The question to be posed is therefore whether any of the three treatments—AM, CBT, or BT—is able to achieve these goals, and if so by what means. Discussion of this question, linking the results described above to these wider characteristics of GAD, can only follow if there is a clearer understanding of what each treatment involves. One cannot devise hypotheses about the mechanism of a treatment without knowing what exactly it entails. Because so little has been written about the treatment of GAD, and because well-known methods (e.g., exposure) may have to be modified for use with this population, these details may also be of interest in their own right.

THREE TREATMENTS FOR GAD

In this section, the three treatments used in the Oxford studies are described and illustrated. It is not possible to provide a comprehensive breakdown of what each involves, but it will aid discussion to set out for each its rationale and the procedures adopted. Despite their apparent complexity, all three of these treatments are held together by simple and clear rationales that can readily be explained. Brief outlines of the treatments are followed by more detailed illustrations of some ways in which they were successful. The intention is to stimulate thinking about specific sources of effectiveness. The first step, however, is to look at the characteristics shared by the different treatments: AM, CBT, and BT.

Shared Characteristics of the Treatments

Although one could look at characteristics that these three treatments share with interventions from other, quite diverse schools, this is a somewhat narrower attempt to look at some characteristics that they share among themselves and that broadly distinguish them from many other approaches. It is important that these characteristics be considered and not dismissed as "nonspecific" factors, since they are likely also to contribute to treatment effectiveness.

The first major aspect that the treatments share is the goal of greater self-control on the part of the patient. To varying degrees, all three treatments are collaborations in which the aim is to foster independence—for example, by having patients learn a set of techniques that helps them to cope with anxiety without resorting either to anxiolytic medication or to overdependence on others.

With self-control as the aim, the preliminary stages of treatment use various strategies—a treatment booklet, the presentation of information about anxiety and of a rationale for treatment, record keeping, and homework—to promote the idea that skills for managing anxiety can be acquired, but have to be learned before they can be applied. These factors provide the framework for a collaborative treatment. They "socialize" the patient and cultivate appropriate expectations: learning to control anxiety rather than seeking to be cured. There is much overlap in the style in which these matters are addressed in the three treatments.

A definite structure, both within each session and over the series of sessions, also characterizes these three approaches. So as to make efficient use of time and clarify what has been learned, procedures such as agenda setting, homework reviews, summaries, and mutual feedback are routinely used during each session. Furthermore, the overall structure of treatment encourages an initial focus on applying the model to the patients' particular problems by way of a detailed formulation. Toward the end of treatment, the aim is shifted toward encouraging patients to take control of the work by systematizing, and thus internalizing, all that they have learned. This process is crystallized by writing out a "blueprint," itself something of a model for independence, before ending treatment. Since relatively little has been written on either of the last two aspects, the ideas behind them are now explained.

Formulations

A formulation provides a way of fitting together the diverse pieces of information provided by patients and a framework within which to draw implications about managing anxiety. It has four main purposes: (1) to explain symptoms, processes, the treatment rationale, why previous coping has not been successful, and so forth; (2) to generate hypotheses—for instance, about maintaining factors, underlying factors, or core beliefs; (3) to put the symptoms into context, so as to identify determining factors or setting conditions for symptoms; and (4) to develop a treatment plan. As a way of conceptualizing the patient's problem, a good formulation should be simple, should aim to account for all the important information given, and should remain open to adaptation in the light of discussion and new information. As used in all three of these treatments, the formulation is thus a dynamic rather than a static tool. It is used as a guide, not a rule, and is shared with the patient rather than kept private. In the most recent of the studies mentioned above (Butler et al., 1991), a detailed formulation was formally discussed with each patient during the fourth session.

The two demands—to account for everything and to provide a simple framework for treatment—may seem to contradict each other. In practice, the method can be used constructively to make sense of the information and the methods discussed during treatment, if the information is carefully structured. A simple framework, such as one distinguishing among predisposing, precipitating, and maintaining factors, can clarify the patient's experience, explain how the therapist understands the problem, and specify the implications of this understanding for treatment. The rationale for treatments based on a "vicious-circle" model of anxiety (common to AM, BT, and CBT), is implicit in this framework, although different implications are drawn and different emphases are given to the parts of the framework in the different treatments. For example, some types of predisposing factors, such as those reflecting beliefs and attitudes, are probably less likely to become clear during BT than during CBT or even AM. Although many patients spontaneously mention that they tend to be worriers, long-standing attitudes such as those reflected in the statements "If I do my best then nothing should go wrong," "I try to please others all the time," and "I'm an all-or-nothing person," are most likely to be mentioned when cognitions are made the main focus of treatment.

Blueprints

Blueprints are intended to crystallize and clarify the aspects of treatment that patients have found helpful, and thus to provide practical guidelines for the future. When improvement occurs in GAD, the diffuse, confusing, and fluctuating nature of the disorder makes it particularly difficult for patients to be clear about what has brought this about. In addition, demoralized patients are less ready to attribute improvement to the success of their own efforts. These problems may be overcome if the methods that people have found useful during treatment are summarized, written down, and retained for future reference. Thus, making a blueprint theoretically clarifies and makes accessible the steps a person has made toward the goal of greater self-control. However, it also serves other functions. It is a way of handing over control to the patient; a reminder that anxiety is normal and therefore will recur; an opportunity to talk about the sorts of events likely to provoke symptoms in the future; a preparation for dealing with setbacks; and a review of treatment.

Examples of blueprint items arising from behavioral procedures are as follows: "Make time for myself and be firm about it," "Don't avoid standing up for myself," and "Decide what my goals are, then it is easier to see how to achieve them (e.g., if the goal is to help M [son] become more independent, then the best way to help him may in fact be to do less for him)." Examples from blueprints summarizing cognitive procedures include the following: "Don't dismiss things, but think them through," "Look for both sides of the question and don't forget to weigh it up," and "Remember these things are harder to do if you feel bad, so if you can't do them it does not show you're stupid, ill, unconfident, unlikeable, bad, etc."

The Three Treatments

Characteristics specific to AM, BT, and CBT are now described; they are also illustrated with examples of their successful application, so as to stimulate thinking about the basis of treatment effectiveness and the processes involved in change. The improvements described all took place within the maximum number of 12 sessions allowed for treatment in these research studies.

Anxiety Management

Description. The rationale for AM is that it is an active, self-help treatment based on a vicious-circle model of anxiety, in which anxiety can be controlled if the factors that maintain it are identified and the vicious circle interrupted. It contains procedures for reducing symptoms (relaxation, distraction, panic management, and controlling upsetting thoughts); graded practice to reduce avoidance; and simple cognitive and behavioral procedures to increase self-confidence and reduce demoralization.

Illustration. After a period of unemployment, an ex-soldier had started a new career as a salesman. He worried about his ability to do the new job; about his health (he had been admitted to a casualty ward after panic attacks on two occasions, and also had a family history of heart disease and a long-standing back injury); and about nearly all his relationships, both at work and at home. He came for treatment in desperation, saying that there was nothing he could do. After his difficulties were discussed in terms of the vicious-circle model, it was agreed to begin with relaxation (partly because of pain in his back and neck, which could result either from tension or from his back injury). He practiced assiduously, found the method helpful, and was able to adapt the methods learned at home so as to apply them during difficult periods at work. In the second session exposure was introduced, as he was avoiding making telephone calls at work. The principles were explained, on the basis that avoidance maintains the problem. Over 4 weeks he successfully increased the daily number of telephone calls, and also identified various more subtle kinds of avoidance of which he was not previously aware, such as not talking to his wife about the problem (for fear of seeming weak), not mentioning difficulties in his job to his boss, and not initiating things at work.

He made good progress working on relaxation and exposure together, until something went wrong at work, when he had a major setback. At this point a cognitive strategy was introduced, as it was clear that he was accepting full responsibility for an event outside his control: "It was all my fault," "I should have been able to prevent this happening," "I shall get the sack." These thoughts were examined using standard cognitive procedures. He finally concluded that he was not responsible for the error in question; rather, it arose because he had "responsibility without the authority to follow things through." As a homework assignment, he raised and resolved this issue with his boss.

Finally, all the strategies used were summarized in a blueprint in as general a way as possible, so that they could be applied in different situations in the future. The reminder that he found most useful was the statement "There *is* something you can do."

Behavior Therapy

Description. The rationale presented for BT is that anxiety is maintained by reactions to symptoms, by avoidance, and by loss of confidence. Since these all interrelate and easily fuel each other, the aim is to prevent a spiraling effect. This is achieved through focusing on behavioral reactions to anxiety, using these as a cue to respond otherwise. The usual maintaining factors of physical tension, avoidance, and loss of confidence are targeted by relaxation, graded exposure, and behavioral methods for increasing confidence.

Illustration. A woman in her 40s had taken up work as a receptionist since her children had left home. She had been tense and worried ever since the children were young, was constantly tired, slept badly, and complained that she was "bothered by everything" (from doing the ironing to her children's future). She felt under pressure and overburdened, had given up reading and seeing friends, and no longer looked forward to weekends. Despite the long history of severe anxiety, her potential to help herself was immediately apparent. She started to work on her problems alone, after reading the treatment booklet and before her first treatment session. She arrived for this session having already drawn up her own target list.

1. *Relaxation.* She learned how to relax quickly, and then turned her attention to applying the technique by shortening the formal exercises, using frequent reminders to check her level of tension, setting aside time to relax and read after lunch, and devising a brief exercise that she could use at work or when doing chores at home. She remarked at the end that she had more energy because she was more relaxed during the day.

2. *Exposure.* From the target list, it was clear that she was avoiding a number of things, but in a typically inconsistent fashion: meeting new people (she did this daily at work); organizing herself ahead of time and stopping to think (she rushed from one task to another for fear of having to face the whole list); "anything that feels like an effort," a phrase that covered almost anything on a bad day; and making telephone calls if she thought she might not be able to handle someone else's irritability or hostility at that time. The principles of exposure were explained, to make sure that she understood that avoidance would maintain the problem and

that she should always face things (if necessary, in a graduated way) rather than avoid them. Instead of planning precise exposure tasks, she kept a record of anything she had, or had specifically not, avoided.

3. *Building confidence and dealing with demoralization.* Pleasures such as walking or seeing friends and relatives had been neglected to the extent that she felt guilty doing even small things for her own pleasure (such as reading a magazine briefly after a meal). These were planned as specific homework tasks. The borderlines among the three different kinds of strategies became increasingly unclear as she improved: for example, making the effort to go out with some women friends (a) made her feel less burdened and isolated, and thus reduced demoralization and increased her sense of being in control; (b) was a step on the way toward asking people in for a meal; and (c) was in itself a relaxing activity—a "recreation" in the true sense of the word.

Once she clearly understood the rationale for treatment, she was, despite her long history, able to build creatively on the general behavioral approach. Additional aspects of the treatment, which she initiated, included organizing herself by planning ahead; identifying and deciding in advance how to handle moments of pressure; setting reasonable housework goals; joining in the community by going to church and contributing to a local traffic census; weekend activities with her husband; planning a holiday to visit her son (living abroad); and, in her own words, "ignoring the irritations" from her husband.

Cognitive–Behavior Therapy

Description. The rationale presented for CBT is that anxiety is maintained by thoughts, whether they be about symptoms, about situations that provoke anxiety, or about self-confidence (or indeed about anything else). The procedure has been laid out clearly in several excellent sources (e.g., Beck et al., 1985; Hawton, Salkovskis, Kirk, & Clark, 1989), though the subtleties involved are often underestimated. At its simplest, the task is for the patient to recognize relevant anxious thoughts, to look for alternatives to them, and to take action to test which accords best with reality.

Behavioral procedures form an integral part of CBT; the tasks are set to test, or collect information relevant to, particular thoughts, attitudes, or beliefs. The results of behavioral homework assignments are thus evaluated in terms of their cognitive implications, but are in other ways similar to those used in both AM and BT. It is therefore to be supposed that the benefits of behavioral procedures contribute to the success of CBT, but that CBT provides additional methods for dealing with thoughts of all kinds, whether they be about primary or secondary problems. The illustrations below are selected so as to emphasize these additional possibilities of CBT.

Illustrations.

1. Reservations about treatment, or beliefs about oneself, may prevent some people from making use of treatment. These people may drop out if the treatment does not tackle these problems directly. For instance, a woman of 34 became anxious and depressed after a succession of life events following the death of her mother 4 years previously. She was an efficient and reliable person to whom others turned for help, and found it difficult to accept that this time she was the one with the problem. She expressed two kinds of thoughts: (a) reservations about coming for treatment, such as "I shouldn't need help," and "Others are far worse off than me"; and (b) self-denigratory or hopeless thoughts about treatment, such as "It's pathetic to be like this," and "If you can't help yourself, there's nothing anyone else can do." She was so reluctant to commit herself to treatment that the first three or four sessions were spent exclusively in dealing with these thoughts. Only after this was she able to devote time and energy to anxiety-related topics.

2. Discussion of thoughts frequently reminds people about earlier, emotionally salient events in their lives that appear to relate to their anxiety states and to pervasive beliefs or attitudes. For example, a young woman had been anxious all her adult life and had recently had to take 3 months off from a training course when her symptoms became worse. After making quite good initial progress, she asked to spend a whole session "telling her life story." This was agreed to, on the understanding that she would take the opportunity to think about how the events of the past were still affecting her in the present. Only after telling the story was she able to put into words the thought, "People with my sort of history can never be confident." After some discussion of this thought, she carried out a homework assignment that involved asking specific other people how they became confident. From this exercise, she learned a number of things that she found helpful: (a) Many people who appear confident are not so underneath; (b) you can be confident about some things but not others; (c) confidence can be acquired—it comes with practice; and there is no need to evaluate yourself poorly because you do not feel confident.

DISCUSSION

Theoretical Background and the Nature of the Disorder

Beck et al. (1985) have elegantly described the goal of treatment for anxiety in terms of achieving a positive or functional balance between perceived demands or threats on the one hand, and perceived resources on the other. As already illustrated, anxious people, and generally anxious ones in particular, perceive threats as many and resources as few. Although there may be some problems for which various approaches appear to restore the equilibrium between the two (at least on a temporary basis), this appears not to be so in the case of GAD. Different approaches may appear to have produced similar outcomes only because their results have been uniformly modest, at least until the last decade (Barrios & Shigetomi, 1979; Rachman & Wilson, 1980; Raskin, Bali, & Peeke, 1980; Rapee, 1991). Very few adequate studies of BT or CBT are available, and the pervasive clinical impression remains that the severe and persistent GAD typical of those patients included in the studies described above remains difficult to treat effectively. It is nevertheless possible that treatments that focus both on reducing the number of perceived threats and on increasing the number of available resources, such as CBT or AM, will be more successful than others. At a superficial level, the illustrations above suggest that BT can be effective when a patient easily adopts the active, self-help approach (one of the characteristics shared by all three treatments described); that AM has the added advantage of simple cognitive methods; and that CBT, being more complex and elaborate, is able to deal more thoroughly with low motivation, blocks in treatment, and underlying beliefs or assumptions. However, this says little about the processes involved in change. In the remainder of this chapter, we examine the determinants of successful outcome in more detail, and consider what the specific elements of successful treatment might be.

At the outset, it is worth re-emphasizing that patients with this disorder describe a bewildering number of diffuse and seemingly uncontrollable thoughts and other symptoms. Because their anxieties have persisted for so long, it may be hard for them to recall what it was like to be free of the problem. Two common and closely linked clinical characteristics are that patients tend to feel overwhelmed, and that they no longer feel able to cope. The consequent demoralization means that they can easily believe that there is indeed nothing they can do about their predicament. Although the opportunity to normalize their fear is an important one, and although techniques such as relaxation may be of some benefit, there is no evidence to suggest that general therapeutic factors such as the former or specific techniques such as the latter will in themselves be of sufficient value to bring about enduring and clinically significant change. In the face of this failure, it may be useful to identify some steps that patients take, or attitudes that they hold, that in our clinical experience seem to provide the setting conditions for change. This is not in any sense an exhaustive list.

Setting Conditions for Change

Perhaps one of the earliest harbingers of progress during treatment for GAD is the extent to which patients are able to respond actively rather than passively to their problem, and to take responsibility for change. A common corollary of helplessness is the expectation that only others can solve the problem. Given the nature of anxiety, such a hope cannot be fulfilled, and it will stand as an important impediment to any treatment based on the self-help model. An essential first step is that patients believe (or quickly come to believe) that a realistic aim is managing rather than eliminating anxiety, and that this is something they can learn to do themselves.

A second, related step is that of problem definition and clarification. GAD sufferers are especially likely to feel overwhelmed by their symptoms and by previous failures to limit or predict them. Faced with such unpredictability and confusion, patients can feel that their problems are more manageable once they have been individually specified and formulated. Providing a formulation based on specific difficulties not only reduces confusion and directs efforts toward self-control strategies, but provides a context within which to present a rationale for treatment. It identifies a firm basis from which energies can be mobilized.

Third, therapists should be aware of what the patients have been trying on their own initiative when explaining specific management strategies. It is often the case that through their own ingenuity or common sense, or that of others, patients have used a variety of commonly proposed techniques. For example, some 80– 90% of subjects in the Oxford studies used several cognitive methods before ever meeting a therapist (Butler, Gelder, et al., 1987). However, they have only rarely found these methods to be effective in controlling anxiety, and have tended to use such techniques inconsistently, when anxiety was too high, or without a clear sense of what to do in particular situations. If the proposed action has not previously been useful, patients may have reservations about trying it again or may be frankly biased against it. If reasons for failure can be found and explained, then the technique can be proposed as an alternative worthy of evaluation, and their interest and involvement are more likely to be secured. Without such engagement, patients may not try to use the specific methods suggested to them during treatment.

If these factors are indeed linked to favorable outcome, one can gain a good sense of why BT has had some degree of success. Some patients may be encouraged by this direct, concise approach to take responsibility for change, to clarify the nature of their problems, and to make good use of their own resources. The patient described in the illustration of BT above seemed to respond to treatment in this way. BT promotes the much-needed clarity and early success that can provide such a boost to confidence. The structure that characterizes BT (as well as AM and CBT) may be particularly important in the treatment of GAD because of the diffuse, pervasive, and confusing nature of the problem. It ensures that the topic being discussed is clear to both parties, that they understand each other well, and that they draw the same conclusions from what they discuss. Clear structuring of treatment sessions provides a model for constructive problem solving. In this sense it is easy to see why BT may facilitate change for those patients who are able to mobilize their own resources in an active and realistic way (so as to control rather than remove symptoms of anxiety). However, the degree of success achieved by BT appears to be limited (Butler et al., 1991; Durham & Turvey, 1987), and in the Butler et al. study attrition rates were unacceptably high (18% in BT, 0% in CBT). A minority became too depressed to continue with treatment, or dropped out for other reasons. Both CBT and AM have proved to be more successful in this and in other respects, the reasons for which require scrutiny.

It seems unlikely that just a single reason will explain why these two approaches are able to go some steps further than BT alone. One possibility is that part of the superiority is accounted for by the relative success of the more cognitive therapies in dealing with the so-called "secondary" problems of GAD—namely, depression, social anxiety, and panic. Though a diagnosis of GAD was not made in our studies if diagnostic criteria were met for these other problems, to lesser degrees they are very much part of GAD. Secondary depression, for example, has been reported in as many as 60% of these patients (see Chapter 6, this volume). From what we know of depression, social anxiety, and panic, we might certainly expect that a cognitive approach would be more potent in dealing with these problems than one focusing exclusively on behavior. This would explain, too, the higher number who drop out of BT, whose hopelessness about the possibility of change has been unchallenged. Put quite simply, BT has fewer options with such secondary problems, and so its results necessarily suffer. It is unlikely, however, that this is the sole difference. Other factors are also likely to be implicated, some of which are now discussed.

In the initial stages of treatment, cognitive approaches allow a full examination of fundamental thoughts about treatment itself and how useful it might be. Cognitive techniques can be readily and effectively deployed to overcome reservations about treatment and low motivation in general. Distortions may be identified that are bringing on a sense of demoralization and that may be so consuming as to obscure positive, adaptive attributes and impede progress. As treatment continues, cognitive approaches allow patient and therapist together to "get a handle" on worry—arguably the key ingredient of the disorder. Most patients require ways of dealing not just with the consequences of anxiety, such as avoidance, loss of confidence, and physical tension, but also with ways of thinking that generate anxiety.

Although it does seem that specific negative thoughts are changed as a result of CBT, it is interesting that in the most recent Oxford study

(Butler et al., 1991) an independent assessor asked each patient at the 6-month follow-up assessment, "What difference has treatment made to the way you deal with anxiety?" It was striking that patients in both groups reported specific factors in their responses, but that those in the CBT group also reported more general factors. They used phrases such as "It puts it in perspective," "I found a way of dealing with it myself," "Instead of it taking me over, I take over it," and "I've made an overall change in my attitude." These phrases imply that the cognitive interventions had done more to bring about a change of attitude in the way patients looked at both their problems and their resources. If so, this would help to explain why the superiority of CBT increased with time. It may also explain why, although it is useful in reducing isolation to hear of other people with the same problem, it takes rather more than this to achieve significant results. It may be that patients not only gain perspective, but go one stage further and learn to cut into a stream of self-criticism and worry.

Two other possibilities should be briefly mentioned. First, during CBT underlying beliefs and assumptions can be discussed and challenged in such a way as (theoretically) to make people less susceptible to future anxiety states. Second, behavioral methods alone may not be sufficient to deal with low self-esteem and poor self-confidence. It appears that some people are able to draw "cognitive conclusions" from behavioral homework assignments without explicit help from a therapist. However, others are not so successful; they may consistently succeed behaviorally, but continue to doubt their abilities and to worry about possible future threats. Clearly, elaborate cognitive methods such as those used in CBT can tackle these difficulties. The apparent success of AM, which employs relatively simple cognitive methods, is less easy to explain. It raises the question as to whether these simple methods, used in the context of a coping rather than a cognitive rationale for treatment, may sometimes be sufficient to potentiate progress and bring about cognitive change. A direct comparison of AM and CBT could well be informative.

Placing These Findings in a Wider Context

Our discussion has thus far deliberately focused on a small group of studies. Casting the net a little wider, we can now ask whether there is support for what has been argued thus far. The answer must of necessity be a little cautious. With such a small literature, it is more accurate to say that there is little to contradict what has been put forward than to say that there is widespread and unequivocal support.

A comprehensive review of psychological treatment studies is not attempted here. Rather, a few relevant points are made. The majority of the (relatively few) studies conducted before the mid-1980s were not carried out with patient subjects but with volunteers. At the same time, the early studies using patients most probably included heterogeneous groups of subjects. Before the improvements made to the definitions of GAD and of panic disorder, it was much harder to make a definite diagnosis; patients with independent or additional diagnoses of panic disorder, hypochondriasis or health anxiety, mild personality disorders, or varying degrees of agoraphobia and social phobia were easily confounded with patients with GAD.

There has been a great improvement in the quality of the studies published more recently, and their findings have been considerably more exciting as the degree of clinically significant change achieved has risen (see above). However, problems still remain. For example, we have as yet no criterion measure of GAD, nor any agreed-upon indicators of clinically relevant improvement; these problems have been solved in different ways by different researchers, and with varying degrees of adequacy. Because the cognitive aspect of GAD is now its main defining feature, measures of relevant cognitions should be, but have not been, used in a standard manner. Making sense of the present research is still therefore a somewhat impressionistic matter.

With these caveats in mind, three points are made here. In the first place, there is sufficient evidence to support the claim that psychological treatments (of various kinds) can achieve more change than would occur spontaneously during a waiting period for patients with relatively severe forms of the disorder (Barlow et al., 1984; Butler, Cullington, et al., 1987; Blowers, Cobb, & Mathews, 1987; Power, Jerrom, Simpson, Mitchell, & Swanson, 1989). Treatment gains also appear to be relatively stable. This in itself is an achievement in a group of people who say that they "have always been worriers" and who have been notoriously difficult to treat.

Second, a number of other studies have reported some superiority for cognitive forms of treatment over other forms (e.g., Durham & Turvey, 1987; Borkovec et al., 1987; Power et al., 1989). For instance, Durham and Turvey (1987) compared BT (including distraction and limited use of positive self-statements) with CBT in a way similar to the Butler et al. (1991) study, previously described at some length. The results are broadly consistent with the latter study, though the effects appear not to have been quite as marked. Thus, while patients in the CBT group did better than those who received BT, even in this group one-third did not show a significant difference from their pretreatment level of functioning. The differences between the two groups were only evident at follow-up, at which point those receiving CBT were maintaining or improving upon their posttreatment gains, whereas many of those receiving BT reverted back to their midtherapy scores. The authors' conclusion was that a cognitive approach is more often able to provide a flexible, widely applicable, and enduring framework for perceiving and coping with problems, very much in accord with the ideas put forward in this chapter. The authors were careful to monitor the quality of the therapy provided, but their results might have been clearer if they had given equivalent attention to differentiating the treatments, given the large number of characteristics they share.

The third point of interest in this context is that nonspecific treatments may be able to achieve gains substantially similar to those achieved by the more specific ones (e.g., Borkovec & Mathews, 1988; Rapee, Adler, Craske, & Barlow, 1988). The results of the Borkovec and Mathews (1988) study may seem quite at odds with the results given earlier. They compared the efficacy of three treatments: nondirective therapy, coping desensitization, and cognitive therapy. Their conclusions were clear, indicating significant improvement on a variety of outcome measures for all subjects, but yet failing to support differential effectiveness among the three therapy conditions. These results need to be explained.

It is possible, for instance, that differences among the treatments were less likely because patients in all three conditions received training in relaxation. However, it may well remain that the results would hold in any case and that an explanation must be sought. The authors conjecture that general factors not linked to any particular approach, such as hope and belief in therapy, may have contributed significantly to change. If so, then this need not be seen as a negative result. Rather, such general factors will need more careful specification, and the question should be raised as to whether treatments that have been shown to be more effective are those in which these general factors have been used most efficiently. However, it may be that the authors' further speculation on how such results might have come about will prove the most interesting. They suggest tellingly that "processes such as alternative conceptualizations of one's anxiety or the self-discovery of coping methods may also be operative" (p. 882). The example they cite is that two of the patients who made the most progress in the nondirective group indicated toward the end of treatment that they "now realized the importance of confronting their fears and of talking more rationally to themselves when they felt anxious." This is consistent with the finding in the Oxford studies that patients spontaneously reported trying to do these things before they received treatment, although initially without much success. It is also consistent with Barlow's suggestion that "any number of psychological treatments may be effective for GAD as a result of positive expectancy, renewed hope, and increased sense of control" (1988, p. 595). As yet we know little about the process of change during successful treatment of GAD. It is intriguing to speculate that similar mechanisms of change may be mobilized in a variety of ways.

Of course, the assumption being made here is that the important factor is to mobilize internal mechanisms of change: to help patients find or learn ways of coping or of managing their anxiety. It would support this assumption to find that treatments that failed to mobilize patients' own resources in either a clear or a creative way, such as using passive rather than active forms of relaxation, achieved a smaller degree of success—a point also made as long ago as 1979 by Barrios and Shigetomi.

Providing passive forms of treatment is only one way of failing to mobilize patients' resources. Failure to achieve this goal may occur for other reasons. For example, treatment packages that combine a number of potentially useful strategies can be more confusing than helpful if they are not also clearly explained (e.g., in the context of a coherent rationale). It has been argued above that the confusing nature of the problem makes this especially important when patients suffer from long-standing GAD. Hence the emphasis placed on the main message "There *is* something you can do" during AM. It is possible that failure to put forward such a clear rationale, and to engage patients in the joint attempt to locate and develop coping resources, accounts for some of the relatively inconclusive findings in the literature—such as those reported by Blowers et al. (1987), in which relatively inexperienced therapists provided two treatments, anxiety management training and nondirective counseling (see also Lindsay, Gamsu, McLaughlin, Hood, & Espie, 1987). If patients receive clear instructions that motivate them to engage with treatment, they seem to be likely to make substantial gains. However, if they receive a nondirective treatment, they appear also to build up their own resources in a creative way to arrive at a not dissimilar point. Is this true? If so, what would it suggest about the processes involved in treatment?

Processes of Change

In simple phobia, a series of steps to bring about change can be recommended; in GAD, by contrast, the path to progress is more blurred and less distinct. Although one might suppose that relaxation would be helpful when someone is feeling tense, that exposure is appropriate when fear leads to avoidance, and that cognitive methods should be used to deal with worry, in practice people may successfully deal with their anxiety by using other methods. This makes it well-nigh impossible to stick to a standardized approach. With such a varied and complex condition, a measure of creativity and a high level of flexibility are required in piecing together a series of steps with a patient. It is perhaps because it is difficult to standardize that the role of creativity has been underplayed and undervalued. A short example will perhaps illustrate that such creativity is neither bland nor straightforward.

The creative elements in therapy may be used for such purposes as identifying coping skills that are already being used, working out how their effectiveness can be maximized, and helping the patient to choose the right skill for the right situation. One particular patient reported using a typically individualized coping strategy. Although they were not of spiritual value for him, he used to handle rosary beads when anxious, and reported that this could alleviate his worry. A careful review of recent occasions on which he had found the beads helpful made it clear that they could serve a number of positive functions. He could use them (although unsystematically) as a form of meditative relaxation, as a means of distraction, as a cue to monitor thoughts, or as a way of generating self-coping statements. By clarifying these different coping methods and by developing associations between particular beads and particular people or themes, he became able to use them even more effectively. However, it also became apparent that there were times when his use of the beads was clearly a subtle avoidant strategy that prevented him from engaging in some form of feared activity. In addition, there was a risk that their constant use might support his belief that he had to have such a prop with him in any situation that he found anxiety-provoking. What was important was (1) that he came to realize that the beads provided a cue to a range of potentially useful coping strategies; (2) that he became more proficient at using them; and (3) that he learned to use them (or not to do so) in the most appropriate way for any particular situation. This one personal strategy, which had originally been of somewhat limited value and which he had at first been embarrassed to describe, was thus developed into a vehicle for discussing and developing coping strategies consistent with the rationale for treatment and comfortably adapted to his personal style. The fact that this was possible served also to increase his self-confidence, as the therapist endorsed his personal method of controlling symptoms and helped him to develop it creatively.

It has not been our purpose in this chapter to argue that cognitive methods provide the only means of developing such an individualized approach, or indeed of treating GAD effectively. Rather, we have suggested that there is good reason to conclude that these methods are promising, and that much can be learned about how else one might tackle GAD by looking closely at processes of change. The suggestion is that being clear, being creative, and boosting confidence (reducing demoralization) are critical elements of successful intervention. They determine the joint ability of patient and therapist to experiment and so adapt to an individual's requirements and resources. These are hardly elements that are restricted to CBT. By comparing different methods—not solely to see which does better, but rather to study the mechanisms and processes of change—this field could progress altogether more quickly. The aim should be not merely to increase the cost-effectiveness of treatment for this disorder, but to learn what leads to successful or to unsuccessful intervention. To this end, it is useful initially to ask what cognitive methods may achieve that behavioral methods may not. Other avenues will be to predict outcome, to study individual differences in response to treatment, and to look more closely at treatment failures. Linking clearly specified treatments to their effects, and noting how, where, and when change occurs, should increase understanding of what is happening. The field is at an early stage for teasing out which of the steps taken by both patient and therapist are required for effective treatment. If this style of analysis has merit, then these tentative suggestions should quickly be superseded.

CONCLUSION

Considering that GAD has been reckoned to be three to four times more common than panic disorder (cited in Barlow, 1988, p. 567; Regier et al., 1988), it is remarkable how little research it has generated. It has been argued that one reason for this is that it has proved so stubborn a condition to treat; only in the last decade have there been grounds for treatment optimism. Now that some progress can be made with this disorder, it is vital to identify what is contributing to this change. Treatment outcome studies may reveal part of the answer, but they have distinct limitations if they merely state that one approach appears to be superior to another. The next, and vital, step is to work out why this should be so; we need models not just of the disorder, but of how change in the disorder takes place. In this chapter, three approaches have been compared in just such an attempt to examine the possible mechanisms of change in GAD. It is not argued that these are the only avenues to the ends achieved, but that much can be gained from careful inspection of clearly defined treatments. As stated at the outset, clarity and creativity on the part of the therapist are called for, both in clinical intervention and in research. Even at this early stage, the results bode well on both fronts when these qualities have been achieved.

REFERENCES

American Psychiatric Association. (1987). *Diagnostic and statistical manual of mental disorders* (3rd ed., rev.). Washington, DC: Author.

Barlow, D. H. (1988). *Anxiety and its disorders: The nature and treatment of anxiety and panic*. New York: Guilford Press.

Barlow, D. H., Cohen, A. S., Waddell, M. T., Vermilyea, B. B., Klosko, J. S., Blanchard, E. B., & Di Nardo, P. A. (1984). Panic and generalized anxiety disorders: Nature and treatment. *Behavior Therapy, 15*, 431–449.

Barrios, B. A., & Shigetomi, C. C. (1979). Coping-skills training for the management of anxiety: A critical review. *Behavior Therapy, 10*, 491–522.

Beck, A. T., Emery, G., & Greenberg, R. (1985). *Anxiety disorders and phobias: A cognitive perspective*. New York: Basic Books.

Beck, A. T., Laude, R., & Bohnert, M. (1974). Ideational components of anxiety neurosis. *Archives of General Psychiatry, 31*, 319–325.

Beck, A. T., Rush, A. J., Shaw, B. F., & Emery, G. (1979). *Cognitive therapy of Depression*. New York: Guilford Press.

Blowers, C., Cobb, J., & Mathews, A. (1987). Generalized anxiety: A controlled treatment study. *Behaviour Research and Therapy, 25*, 493–502.

Borkovec, T. D. (1985). Worry: A potentially valuable concept. *Behaviour Research and Therapy, 23*, 481–482.

Borkovec, T. D., & Hu, S. (1990). The effect of worry on cardiovascular response to phobic imagery. *Behaviour Research and Therapy, 28*, 69–73.

Borkovec, T. D., & Inz, J. (1990). The nature of worry in generalized anxiety disorder: A predominance of thought activity. *Behaviour Research and Therapy, 28*, 153–158.

Borkovec, T. D., Mathews, A. M., Chambers, A., Ebrahimi, S., Lytle, R., & Nelson, R. (1987). The effects of relaxation training with cognitive therapy or nondirective therapy and the role of relaxation-induced anxiety in the treatment of generalized anxiety. *Journal of Consulting and Clinical Psychology, 55*, 883–888.

Borkovec, T. D., & Mathews, A. M. (1988). Treatment of nonphobic anxiety: A comparison of nondirective, cognitive, and coping desensitization therapy. *Journal of Consulting and Clinical Psychology, 56*, 877–884.

Butler, G. (1985). Exposure as a treatment for social phobia: Some instructive difficulties. *Behaviour Research and Therapy, 223*, 651–657.

Butler, G., and Anastasiades, P. (1988). Predicting response to anxiety management in patients with generalized anxiety disorder. *Behaviour Research and Therapy, 26*, 531–534.

Butler, G., Cullington, A., Hibbert, G., Klimes, I., & Gelder, M. (1987). Anxiety management for persistent generalized anxiety. *British Journal of Psychiatry, 151*, 535–542.

Butler, G., Cullington, A., Munby, M., Amies, P., & Gelder, M. (1984). Exposure and anxiety management in the treatment of social phobia. *Journal of Consulting and Clinical Psychology, 52*, 642–650.

Butler, G., Fennell, M., Robson, P., & Gelder, M. (1991). A comparison of behavior therapy and cognitive behavior therapy in the treatment of generalized anxiety disorder. *Journal of Consulting and Clinical Psychology, 59*, 167–175.

Butler, G., Gelder, M., Hibbert, G., Cullington, A., & Klimes, I. (1987). Anxiety management: Developing effective strategies. *Behaviour Research and Therapy, 25*, 517–522.

Durham, R. C., & Turvey, A. A. (1987). Cognitive therapy vs. behaviour therapy in the treatment of chronic general anxiety: Outcome at discharge and at six month follow-up. *Behaviour Research and Therapy, 25,* 229–234.

Hawton, K., Salkovskis, P., Kirk, J., & Clark, D. (1989). *Cognitive behaviour therapy for psychiatric problems: A practical guide.* Oxford: Oxford University Press.

Hibbert, G. (1984). Ideational components of anxiety: Their origin and content. *British Journal of Psychiatry, 144,* 618–624.

Jannoun, L., Oppenheimer, C., & Gelder, M. (1982). A self-help treatment program for anxiety state patients. *Behavior Therapy, 13,* 103–111.

Lindsay, W. R., Gamsu, C. V., McLaughlin, E., Hood, E. M., & Espie, C. A. (1987). A controlled trial of treatments for generalized anxiety. *British Journal of Clinical Psychology, 26,* 3–16.

Power, K. G., Jerrom, D. W. A., Simpson, R. J., Mitchell, M. J., & Swanson, V. A. (1989). A controlled comparison of cognitive-behaviour therapy, diazepam and placebo in the treatment of generalized anxiety. *Behavioural Psychotherapy, 17,* 1–14.

Rachman, S., & Wilson, T. (1980). *The effects of psychological therapies.* Oxford: Pergamon Press.

Rapee, R. M. (1985). Distinctions between panic disorder and generalized anxiety disorder: Clinical presentations. *Australian and New Zealand Journal of Psychiatry, 19,* 227–232.

Rapee, R. M. (1991). Generalized anxiety disorder: A review of clinical features and theoretical concepts. *Clinical Psychology Review, 11,*

Rapee, R. M., Adler, C., Craske, M., & Barlow, D. H. (1988, September). *Cognitive restructuring and relaxation in the treatment of generalized anxiety disorder: A controlled study.* Paper presented at the World Congress of Behaviour Therapy, Edinburgh.

Raskin, M., Bali, L., & Peeke, H. (1980). Muscle feedback and transcendental meditation. *Archives of General Psychiatry, 37,* 93–97.

Regier, D. A., Boyd, J. H., Burke, J. D., Rae, D. S., Myers, J. K., Kramer, M., Robins, L. N., George, L. K., Karno, M., & Locke, B. Z. (1988). One-month prevalence of mental disorders in the United States. *Archives of General Psychiatry, 45,* 977–986.

Suinn, R. M., & Richardson, F. (1971). Anxiety management training: A nonspecific behavior therapy program for anxiety control. *Behavior Therapy, 2,* 498–510.

York, D., Borkovec, T. D., Vasey, M., & Stern, R. (1987). Effects of worry and somatic anxiety induction on thought intrusions, subjective emotion, and physiological activity. *Behaviour Research and Therapy, 25,* 523–526.

Index